NATURAL CHILDBIRTH THE SWISS WAY

D1565969

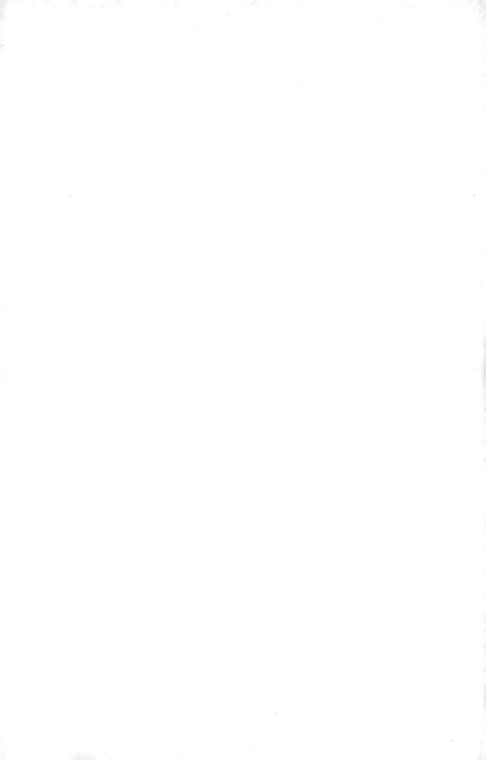

NATURAL CHILDBIRTH THE SWISS WAY

Esther Marilus

PRENTICE-HALL, INC., Englewood Cliffs, N.J.

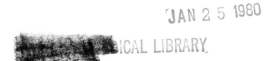

Natural Childbirth the Swiss Way by Esther Marilus
Copyright© 1979 by Esther Marilus
Printed in the United States of America
Prentice-Hall International, Inc., London
Prentice-Hall of Australia, Pty. Ltd., Sydney
Prentice-Hall of Canada, Ltd., Toronto
Prentice-Hall of India Private Ltd., New Delhi
Prentice-Hall of Japan, Inc., Tokyo
Prentice-Hall of Southeast Asia Pte. Ltd., Singapore
Whitehall Books Limited, Wellington, New Zealand
10 9 8 7 6 5 4 3 2 1

Library of Congress Cataloging in Publication Data
Marilus, Esther
   Natural childbirth the Swiss way.
   1. Natural childbirth.   I. Title.
RG661.M36   618.4'5   78-9952
ISBN 0-13-610055-4
ISBN 0-13-610048-1 (pbk)

CONTENTS

To my own mother, Ruth Amsel Thumim,
who, like so many women of her time
was denied the beauty and challenge of
a natural childbirth, and to Itzchak,
my husband and my mainstay
during the writing of this book.

ACKNOWLEDGEMENTS

So many doctors, therapists, gymnasts, and of course mothers have contributed to the quality of today's Swiss prenatal exercise classes, that it would be impossible to mention them all—even if I knew who they were. Nevertheless, I would like to thank sincerely those who personally contributed to the quality of my own training. They are: Dr. H. U. Häfner, who was my instructor at a course given for maternity gymnastic students at the Maternité Inselhof of Triemli Hospital in Zurich; Dr. Nurit Lowinger, who was always ready and able to answer any medical questions that arose during the writing of this book; and Mrs. R. Menne, gymnast and well-known pioneer and teacher in the field of maternity gymnastics, who held a seminar for maternity gymnasts in Zurich, which I was fortunate to attend.

I am also indebted to:

Dr. G. Krebs, advocate of graduated breathing and well-known veteran in the field of childbirth education, for his cooperation and encouragement.

Mrs. C. Schechter, gymnast and friend, for her assistance with the selection of exercises.

Mrs. S. DePaulmsieux, physical therapist at the Red Cross hospital where all of my children were born, who offered her time and expertise to help me put together a comprehensive, step-by-step postpartum routine.

Lisa Collier, whose insight and enthusiasm are responsible for bringing this method to the American public.

Rose Weiner, my spirited cousin and childhood friend, who spent many tiring hours patiently listening to and commenting on the unpublished manuscript from her hospital bed.

Brigitte Muller, our real-life Mary Poppins, who propitiously entered our home in time to rescue me from diapering, feeding, refereeing, and picking up after four children as I raced to meet my approaching deadline.

Thank you, too, to Oscar Collier, my editor, for his efforts, his support and his genuine interest in furthering this method in the United States; to my sister-in-law, Pessy Marilus, who drew many of the anatomical sketches; to Gabrielle Kocherhans, the charming model who graces the photographs; and to Audrey Haas, who typed the manuscript.

Special thanks to Dina Spira, my sister, who offered hospitality, constructive criticism, and free child-care services to my children while I did research for this book during my recent visit to New York. And to Shava Jafee, my "little" sister, who made it all possible by daring to experiment with a different way of birth.

I am also indebted to the many American childbirth educators who compared notes with me, and in some instances allowed me to visit their classes, so that I might see for myself the differences between preparing for childbirth in the United States and in Switzerland. I am indebted as well to Dr. Max Lilling, who arranged for me to witness natural childbirth in a progressive American hospital.

Most of all I would like to express my deepest gratitude to my energetic 70-year-young teacher, Mrs. Edith Risch, who first prepared me for natural childbirth and who, as founder and former president of the Swiss Society for Professional Maternity Gymnasts, has greatly advanced the standards and popularity of Swiss prenatal exercise classes. Every instructor has her own individual approach, making each class somewhat different from the others, and I was fortunate to have studied and worked under the tutelage of an expert, whose enthusiastic teaching style comes close to being an art.

In passing this method on to others, either in person or through this book, I have tried to convey what I have learned just as I learned it; these teachings nevertheless allow a small margin for flexibility and growth and are tempered by my personal experience, both as a mother and as an instructor who has tried, tested, and taught the Swiss way over and over again.

FOREWORD

by Ilva Oehler, M.D.

Not long after the publication of his book *Childbirth Without Fear*,* Grantly Dick-Read lectured on the subject to an audience of gynecologists at the Frauenklinik hospital in Zurich. I still vividly recall his ardent fervor in introducing us to his new method, and the impression left on me by his wife's enthusiastic remark, "Love is wonderful—but childbirth is divine!" A very bold statement in those days.

Only hesitantly and with a trace of reluctance did a group of independent gynecologists and remedial gymnasts undertake to put together a more or less uniform prenatal exercise program based on his theory. Ironically, the German translation of Dr. Read's book, entitled *Die Schmerzlos Geburt* (*Painless Childbirth*), proved more of a hindrance to their work than an asset, since many of the women who read it expected to be "rewarded" for exercising during pregnancy with a totally painless childbirth—and were ultimately disappointed.

For this reason, Dr. Thomas Rust wrote his own book in 1956 on a combined physical and mental approach to childbirth and named it simply, *Die Natürliche Geburt* (*Natural Childbirth*). Consequently, local gynecologists lecturing in Zurich to pregnant women and their husbands placed more and more emphasis on relaxation techniques and on the positive, human aspects of an actively experienced childbirth.

When some gymnastic teachers, trained in the Lamaze school of childbirth preparation, incorporated the Lamaze method in their prenatal gymnastic classes, it soon became apparent to many of us who assisted during labor that this

*In which he emphasized the need for prenatal exercises.

method, with its use of superficial breathing during the first stage of labor, often led to undesirable side effects. It seemed that very few of the women trained in this way were able to master the breathing techniques well enough to avoid hypoxaemia and respiratory alkalosis through hyperventilation. Consequently, we in the field of obstetrics were glad to see an increasing number of young gymnastic instructors beginning to teach a graduated type of deep breathing which enhanced physical relaxation and greatly reduced the chances of hyperventilation tetany during labor.

Today, even in many of the larger hospitals (where skepticism prevailed at first), prenatal exercises have gained recognition and maternity gymnastics are the accepted norm—despite the initial opposition of veteran midwives, who were compelled to forgo their age-old practice of strict, authoritarian rule for the more comforting and persuading ways of the modern midwife.

Since the late 1950's this combined approach for preparing for natural childbirth has, to some extent, been accepted almost everywhere in Switzerland. And although there are no existing statistics to prove it, the overall impression definitely is: that preparing for natural childbirth through physical exercises and the proper breathing and relaxation techniques does significantly ease and expediate childbirth.

PREFACE

by Hans Sauter, M.D., Priv. Doz.

When Esther Marilus chose the title *Natural Childbirth the Swiss Way,* it was with the intent of emphasizing that the instructions given do not adhere rigidly to any one basic method, but have evolved gradually in Switzerland—the results of years of close collaboration between doctors and gymnastic teachers. Today, having stood the test of experience, these procedures have proved to be of definite benefit to the expectant mother.

The descriptions of the gymnastic exercises, their goals, and how they are to be performed, are, I feel, very well presented. The light, humorous undertones also help make this book enjoyable to read and easy to comprehend. Of particular significance, and worthy of praise, is the author's repeatedly drawing attention to the fact that the choice of exercises, positions assumed during labor, and above all else, the choice of breathing techniques should be left to the individual. *They* should be adapted to the personal needs of the mother during *her* pregnancy and labor and not the other way around!

This book will undoubtedly help make natural childbirth a more pleasant experience for many women and will also show them the way to care safely and effectively for themselves—their physical well-being and appearance—during the taxing months of pregnancy.

A PERSONAL INTRODUCTION: MY OWN STORY

As I marched around the gym in time to the beat of a tambourine, kicking my legs up higher than I ever thought I could, swinging my hips, and exercising every muscle in my pregnant body, I felt myself growing a little bit lighter, a little bit taller, and delightfully loose all over. This certainly wasn't what I had expected of a natural childbirth class! But then this was Switzerland, not my native New York, and everything about the country—the people, my pregnancy, and the very idea of having a really "natural" childbirth—was new and exciting.

I had come here at the suggestion of my obstetrician, who believed that these exercises would improve my chances for an easier birth and a speedier recovery. I continued to come, week in and week out, throughout my entire pregnancy, because I liked the way these exercises made me feel; I was swept along by the intense enthusiasm of the class and fascinated by the sheer stamina and vitality that radiated from my 60-year-old teacher. But I didn't fully appreciate the natural childbirth training I received at my "Schwangerschafts Gymnastik" course until years later, when I tried to give birth without it. . . .

Because my first child had been born so swiftly (within two and a half hours of labor) and with so little pain, I came to conclude that the pains of childbirth were grossly exaggerated and that natural childbirth, with or without the bother of conscious relaxation and controlled breathing, was not such a big feat after all. Consequently, when the time came for my second child to be born, I called our babysitter, kissed my "big" boy good-bye, and left cheerfully, eagerly, for the hospital—determined not to bother with most of the breathing techniques or the self-hypnotic relaxation I had used before.

Of course I did relax, in the usual sense of the word, as I lay on my side (in the position commonly used in Europe), chatting with my husband and the midwife between contractions. And whenever a contraction became too intense to ignore, I would quickly take a deep cleansing breath and then low-pant over it (although I had learned not to use this form of breathing unless all else failed). Nevertheless, I was definitely *not* in a state of trancelike relaxation, preoccupied with catching each and every contraction at its start. I reasoned that I didn't have to bother with all that since I wasn't afraid and therefore couldn't "tense up" and cause myself "real" pain. Besides, considering how short my first labor had been, I felt certain that it would soon be over.

Yet three hours later I was still only three fingers dilated. My doctor ruptured the membranes and left—for supper. At that point my spirits began to sink while my contractions reached new, unimaginable heights of intensity. Within minutes they had become really vicious, attacking on three fronts: in front, in back, and running up the insides of my thighs.

Lying on the hard hospital bed, I began to toss from side to side in agony, waiting only to jump up, to fight, to climb the walls and escape the sharp teeth of my contractions as they dug into me again and again, tightening their grip with each blow.

In desperation I tried one breathing technique after another. They helped somewhat. But not enough! I was definitely sinking; yet I fought to hang on, to see it through to the ecstatic climax I knew birth to be. But how? I was clearly beyond attaining a state of deep relaxation. Yet surely, something else, some "trick" or position I'd learned could still help me.

Only one came to mind.

Doubtful if it would work, but unable to remain lying any longer, I flung my cover aside, sat up, turned over, and knelt down on my hands and knees. Oh, what relief! That miserable, wrenching pressure gnawing at my back was eased—practically gone! I could hear water (leaking from me?) running down my legs onto the sterile sheets, the doctor's chair, and all the way down to the floor. Who cared? I had the upper hand now and nothing else mattered.

I raised my forearms off the bed, rested my face in the palms of my hands, closed my eyes, and tried to let go-o-o, as I slowly inhaled up . . . up . . . up . . . . and over . . . . my contraction wave.

This time it worked, and I felt perfectly content to remain just as I was for hours, if necessary.

It wasn't. Within minutes the matronly midwife returned to check my progress. Mumbling something incoherent about Americans and yoga, she turned me gently but firmly back down on my side. I offered no resistance or explanations, not wanting to interrupt my relaxation and risk plummeting down once more into the abyss of pain that I had only barely managed to escape. Instead, I continued to breathe quietly and peacefully over my contractions.

Twenty *bearable* minutes later, I felt that long-awaited urge to push. I wanted to laugh for joy. My baby was coming! My husband rushed out to call the midwife while I "low-panted" like a lioness to keep myself from pushing too soon.

From that point on everything went very quickly. My bed was raised to a leaning-back, sitting position, my legs were put up into stirrups, and I was given the green light to push. I gave one good, satisfying P-U-S-HHhhh for the head to crown, and then stopped short on command to let my doctor work the head out and quickly slip off the cord which was wrapped twice around my baby's neck. Then, after two more half-strength pushes I sat back and watched, in utter fascination, as my second son slowly materialized before my very eyes, casting a spell—an aura of wonder—over us all. I held my breath as he gracefully unfolded, like a Japanese lantern, opening his twinkling little eyes and looking peacefully around—completely unperturbed—before breaking the spell with one short unenthusiastic "wah." Impulsively I reached down to touch him and caught a glimpse of what love is all about.

The cord was cut and he was taken to be bathed. I leaned back on my pillow, physically spent but tingling all over with a happiness and satisfaction that transcended words. The clock on the wall read 7:58 P.M. Only 4 hours and 52 minutes had elapsed since I first entered the hospital, but at least one of those hours had been the longest and hardest of my life. Never again, I vowed, would I doubt the words—and real anguish—of women who suffered during childbirth, but neither would I ever again remain helpless and vulnerable in the face of my own contractions. I wanted childbirth both ways: natural and bearable. And with the help of God and my versatile Swiss training, I knew it was possible.

Today, after two more Swiss-style natural childbirths, I strongly believe that other American women should be given the chance to benefit from the same intense, all-round training I received at my "Schwangerschafts Gymnastik" classes. To be sure, there are many methods of "prepared" (not necessarily natural) childbirth training in the United States, but the overall emphasis is clearly on the psychological rather than the physiological aspects of preparation. Yet childbirth is, first and foremost, a biological function which, although inspiring, can be painful if the mother does not have the know-how and the sheer physical stamina to cope with her contractions. For this reason the invigorating physical exercises taught in Switzerland are just as much an integral part of the training as, say, controlled breathing techniques.

Of course, every method of childbirth training has been known to work—for some. But the Swiss method* makes childbirth so much easier—and so much calmer—even during transition. A woman using this method does not have to work so hard to overcome her contractions, and her baby's oxygen supply is not threatened by shallow, rapid, chest breathing. On the contrary, by cutting down on all conscious physical activity and breathing adequately, but not excessively, during labor, she increases the circulation to and from her uterus (and her baby!). What's more, the mother *feels* better during pregnancy, during childbirth, and after.

The only disadvantage of the Swiss way to natural childbirth is that it takes time to learn. But then, it takes nine months to have a baby. . . .

*A term I have coined to differentiate the training I received in Switzerland and the methods taught in the United States.

PROLOGUE
ONE CASE HISTORY: The Swiss Method Goes to New York

When my sister was lying in labor with her second child, some of the nurses on the floor thought she was sleeping and one even suspected that her contractions (which were being intravenously induced by pitocin*) had stopped.

She wasn't asleep; and her contractions hadn't stopped. It just seemed that way, because she was employing the Swiss method of natural childbirth in a New York City hospital—and none of the nurses had ever seen anything like it before.

Instead of staring, whistling, stroking her abdomen, turning her head rhythmically from side to side to the beat of her controlled breathing, and tapping out a tune on her thigh,† as she had done during her first attempt (and failure) at natural childbirth, she was lying quietly on her side, eyes closed and body limp, yet mentally "tuned in" to herself, ready for her next contraction. When she felt one coming, she would sigh softly and then slowly "breathe over" it by doing one of the three soothing, "graduated" breathing techniques she had learned, all the while picturing her uterus at work opening up the door-out-to-life for her baby.

Because she was breathing slowly through her nose, she never suffered the exhaustion, the dryness, and the hyperventilation she had known with her first childbirth. Like every other woman prepared in this unique method, she knew to "save" the more difficult "open-mouth" breathing techniques she had learned for those really hard contractions at the end of the first stage of labor. (It was reassuring to know that she

---

*An artificial stimulant used to induce labor and to intensify the frequency and strength of contractions.

† The distraction tactics she had learned at a Lamaze School of childbirth preparation.

had them in reserve, just in case.) But before she ever felt the need to use them, she had reached full dilation and was being wheeled into the delivery room.

How do I know? I was there, not as a coach, but as a companion and observer. I wanted to *see* for myself if the method that had worked so well for me and thousands of other women in Switzerland could work as well for an American mother in a New York hospital. I also wanted to know if her using the Swiss method instead of the one she had used before would make a significant difference. I had been told by several American childbirth educators that it would not, that it did not really matter which method a woman used as long as she believed in it and in herself. These experts asserted that it was the general lack of encouragement, if not outright opposition, that the American mother often encountered at the hospital—and not any specific method—that made natural childbirth so much harder, and rarer, in America than it is in Switzerland.

Indeed, right from the start my sister did encounter opposition! When the mother is lying down, the Swiss method calls for curling up comfortably on the side, with the spine curved. But until her doctor came to her rescue, the first nurse on duty absolutely refused to let her turn from her back to her side (a change which increases the maternal circulation by at least 20 percent*).

Nevertheless, despite the initial aggravation with the nurse, the nerve-wracking cries from other women in the ward, the fetal monitor strapped around her belly, the intravenous injection stuck in her arm, the mounting intensity of her induced contractions, and her well-grounded fears (based on painful experience in that very same hospital), my sister was able to maintain a deep trancelike state of relaxation and, to put it in her own words: "To feel the pressure, but stay above the pain."

---

*Ken Ueland, M.D., and John Hansen, M.D., "Maternal Cardiovascular Dynamics, Posture and Uterine Contractions," *American Journal of Obstetrics and Gynecology*, Vol. 1 (1969).

At exactly 1:42 P.M. my little niece was born (à la Leboyer), only 3 hours and 23 minutes after the first induced contraction—not an unusually short labor for a woman trained in the Swiss method.

For my sister and her husband the joy, the thrill, and the overwhelming beauty of natural childbirth was a totally new, peak experience, to be cherished and shared for life. They also had that extra satisfaction of having gambled and won. They had opted for a method of childbirth that was totally unknown to their doctor and never used by their friends . . . and it did make a difference!

I.

PHYSICAL FITNESS FOR THE MOTHER-TO-BE

AUTHOR'S NOTE

The choice of shapely models was meant to spur the expectant reader on to work toward achieving similar contours and to remind her that these exercises should be started before she looks obviously pregnant. Using non-pregnant models also makes it easier to see many of the subtle body movements involved.

Chapter One

PRE-NATAL EXERCISE: WHY, WHEN, AND HOW?

Preparing for childbirth is not enough! You also need to watch out for the "wear and tear" of pregnancy, as any mother who has ever struggled to regain her former figure and vitality can verify. Childbirth passes within hours, but many of the "normal" discomforts of pregnancy are the beginnings of lifelong muscular problems. What's more, as gratifying as an active, participating childbirth can be, the experience is even better when you can leave the hospital in your prepregnancy clothes.

So don't wait until after your baby is born to start exercising your way back into form. If you do, you may discover, too late, that muscles which have been stretched and strained for nine months have lost much of their former elasticity. You may also find that some of the side effects of pregnancy (varicose veins, backache, and so on) don't simply disappear with the baby's arrival. Be realistic. If you normally need to exercise to keep fit (and who doesn't), then you certainly need to do so during pregnancy—a period literally riddled with physical pitfalls. Done regularly, from the fourth month on, these carefully selected exercises also help keep you physically fit for childbirth, a most strenuous physical activity.

Check with your doctor before you begin any exercises. Once you have his okay, you can plan your own exercise routines by following programs A and B (see chapters 2 and 3) in sequence, doing one complete program each day. When you've mastered the basics of good posture and become fairly accomplished in the exercises of these two programs, you're ready to add a mix 'n' match program to your choice of daily workouts. Just follow the sample program charted on page 25, or if you like, put together your own exercise routine by mixing and matching from the various exercises given in Part I of this book, always taking care to exercise from head to toe.

For best results time yourself when you work out. For good, effective training you need to exercise for 15–20 minutes a day (or at least every other day), always including some squatting and pelvic floor exercises. And, of course, if you have reason to suspect that you're a candidate for varicose veins, then you'll have to stick to the anti-varicosity program as well.

To help you in your daily vigil, turn on the music and get your husband (or some other good friend) to join you. You'll know it was worth the effort when you catch a glimpse of yourself pushing that baby carriage proudly down the street. Your baby won't be all that you'll be proud of.

CHARTING AN ALL-ROUND EXERCISE PLAN

Besides your regular daily workout you should get into the habit of exercising your legs every morning before getting out of bed. Do the three simple waking-up exercises (found in Chapter 1) that help guard against varicose veins and other circulatory complications. All together they take less than 4 minutes of your time.

In addition to this, make it a point to exercise your undercarriage at different times of the day and to squat whenever you need to bend down.

If your mother (like mine) has varicose veins and/or your legs feel heavy, consider yourself a candidate for this all-too-common side-effect of pregnancy and invest a few minutes more each day for carrying out the complete anti-varicosity program outlined in Chapter 4.

To help you plan a daily exercise routine that meets all of your needs from head to toe, study the following exercise chart.

RECOMMENDED DAILY EXERCISE CHART

EXERCISES	WHEN	EXTRAS FOR VARICOSE VEIN CANDIDATES
Three waking-up anti-varicosity exercises	Lying in bed in the morning	Repeat 1-2 times, preferably during the afternoon and again at night
The daily workout		
Choose one of the basic programs given, or put together your own mix 'n' match program	Whenever convenient; except after meals	Take a break during the day to do Part B of the anti-varicosity program
Note: Don't start mixing 'n' matching until you've become familiar with the basics of programs A and B.		
Squatting	Any time, whenever you get the chance, and whenever you need to pick something up, cut toenails, etc.	Don't squat down for long. If you have varicose veins, use the sitting position whenever possible
Pelvic floor training Pelvic tilting exercises Stop and go exercises	At every opportunity: while watching TV, washing dishes, etc.	

Note: 15–20 minutes of exercises is the minimum daily requirement. More is fine, if you feel up to it, providing you follow instructions, watch your breathing, and take time to rest in between exercises.

SAMPLE HEAD-TO-TOE MIX 'N' MATCH WORKOUT

EXERCISES	DO	PAGE
The warming-up walk	After posture check, walk for 1 minute, include all extras	44
One-legged knee-bends	5 bends on alternate sides	47
Bent-knee swings	5 back-and-forth swings with each leg	48
Kick-up	3 kicks with each leg	49
Leg twister	Twist and untwist each extended leg 3-4 times	50
The stilted walk	8 steps standing, 10 walking	51
The back-to-wall or free standing spinal roll (followed up with a quick fist massage)	2-3 times, moving very slowly and pausing in between	39
The criss-cross arm stretch	2 times	54
The bosom bounce	Standing, 10 bounces with arms at shoulder level and 10 more with arms in front of nose	59
The leaning-back pelvic rock	8 back-and-forth rocks	35
The sitting squat	2 times	79
Waistline tucks	5 tucks on each side	75
The side-lying shrug	8 stretch-shrug movements with each leg	75
The merry-go-round stretch	3 rounds in either direction	67
Leg-swinging spinal twists	8-10 back-and-forth swings	68
The torso tilt	3-5 times	70
The lying-down spine stretch	2 times, followed by spine-swinging	37
The half-way curl-up	4-5 times	72
The side-twist curl-up	2 times	72
The one-legged twist	6 twists lying down and 10 twists sitting	73
Upside-down scissors	Once	90
Spine rolling	2 times, followed by spine-swinging	92

End by resting on your side, with legs bent and drawn up, elbows flexed and eyes closed. Breathe quietly according to your own natural rhythm. When you feel ready, rise slowly in stages and open your eyes.

GUIDELINES FOR EXERCISING DURING PREGNANCY

Not so long ago a pregnant woman regarded herself as being in a very delicate state. Today the pendulum has swung in the opposite direction. For many young mothers-to-be, anything goes from yoga to belly dancing.

Clearly, both attitudes can be carried to extremes. While pregnancy is not a sickness, it *is* a condition which brings about certain physiological changes and the added responsibility of caring for another human life plus its highly complex, life-sustaining organ—the placenta. These factors set the pregnant woman apart from her nonpregnant contemporaries.

Nevertheless, in the United States, where physical fitness has only recently come of age (an estimated 60 million adult Americans now do some form of regular exercise), finding an exercise class geared to the special needs of the expectant mother is difficult. Even the few that profess to do so are often taught by instructors with no training in the field of maternity gymnastics. More often than not, the expectant American mother in search of a good once-a-week exercise class ends up in a regular gymnastic class, acting under the assumption that as long as you feel fine, anything goes.

"Not so!" say Swiss physicians and maternity gymnasts. Certain otherwise harmless movements can be hazardous during pregnancy. To help you know just where to draw the line when exercising, here are some sound guidelines:

1. Always exercise in a well-ventilated room. Your need for oxygen is greater during pregnancy.
2. Pay attention to your breathing as you exercise and give yourself time to breathe deeply in between exercises.
3. When lying flat on your back, never lift or lower your outstretched legs simultaneously, and never lift one leg while the other is stretched out flat. This could place too great a strain on lower back and abdominal muscles and on the round ligaments anchoring the uterus in place in front. Instead, if you want to raise one leg, first draw up the knee of

the other leg at a 45-degree angle, and keep the bent knee in place until after lowering your raised leg. To draw up both knees, bend first one knee and then the other—never both at once. To lower, straighten first one knee and then the other.

4. When torso is erect and/or legs are straight, never stretch both arms up overhead or bend backwards. This could result in premature separation of the placenta from the uterine wall. To play it safe, leave *all* "reach-to-your-outer-limit" stretches out of your daily routine.

5. Should you feel faint while lying flat on your back, turn quickly over on your side and breathe naturally until the feeling is overcome.

6. When turning from your back to your side or from side to side, draw up your knees and support your enlarged abdomen by literally "holding" it with your arms and hands, as illustrated in Figure 1-1.

7. When going from a supine to a sitting position or vice versa, always wrap one arm around your belly for support, draw up your knees and leaning to one side, prop your weight on your elbow, as illustrated in Figures 1-2 and 1-3.

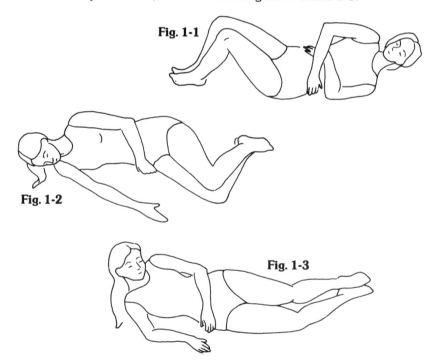

Fig. 1-1

Fig. 1-2

Fig. 1-3

8. Never rise abruptly after exercising. Take your time. Curl up comfortably on your side and breathe quietly for a moment or two. Then do some good, lazy stretching. Yawn if you can and slowly sit up before rising in stages, first on one foot and then on the other.

WARNING
1. **Don't do any pelvic-tilting exercises if you have a sound medical reason for suspecting premature labor.**
2. **Don't do any squatting exercises if you have an incompetent internal os (better known as a "loose cervix") or if you have had an amputation of the cervix or a Shirokar operation.**

BASIC BREATHING INSTRUCTIONS

1. If you are to get the most out of an exercise, with a minimum of fatique, every movement should correspond and harmonize with your breathing. Unless otherwise specified, the rule to remember is this: *Exhale as you tense your muscles,* and *inhale as you relax them.*
2. Never force your inhalations. Doing so could interfere with the natural oxygen-carbon dioxide balance of your body and might result in hyperventilation (which means a lack of

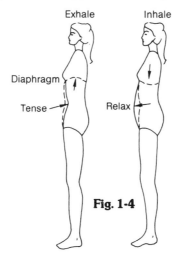

Exhale   Inhale

Diaphragm

Tense   Relax

Fig. 1-4

oxygen in the blood reaching your baby). To lengthen and deepen your inhalations, just exhale somewhat forcefully to push all the air out of your lungs. Then wait, and let breathing in take care of itself. The amount of air you inhale will be automatically determined by your *need* for oxygen, or in other words, by the amount of air you exhaled.

3. When an exercise starts on an inhale, precede it with a deep exhalation.

4. For those exercises which call for prolonged exhalations, inhale through the nose and exhale through the mouth by blowing out softly with a slight hissing sound: *sssssss*. Otherwise breathe through your nose.

Chapter Two

PROGRAM A

PREGNANCY VERSUS POSTURE _____

Pregnancy can run havoc with your posture—if you let it! So take precautions: exercise and watch your posture for flaws at all times. Remember that posture is essential to good looks.

No matter how perfect your posture was before, chances are that as the weight of your baby increases, you will gradually give way to the extra load within your pelvis by tilting it forward, baby and all, assuming a leaning-back, belly-forward, bottom-out stance. Besides adding inches to your waist and bottom, such a typically pregnant posture throws an even greater strain on your already stretched abdominal muscles, as the weight of the baby is thrown forward out of the bony pelvic basin where it belongs and into the soft ab-

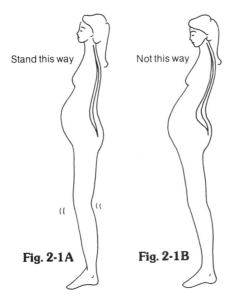

Stand this way   Not this way

Fig. 2-1A   Fig. 2-1B

dominal tissues. Poor posture also puts an unnecessary strain on many of the ligaments and muscles in the lower back, often causing the well-known backache of pregnancy. What's more, poor posture can become a habit that leads to inverted thighs, troublesome feet, poor circulation, stiffness in neck and shoulders, a droopy bosom, stooped shoulders, depressed ribs (which in turn leads to inadequate breathing), and tension all along the spinal column. Considering the consequences, doesn't it make sense to make a conscious all-out effort to sit, stand, and walk correctly, with a minimum of stress and strain on your body?

Here are some tried and proven exercises for developing an automatic postural sense. They will also help to keep your spine and joints flexible and to strengthen the many muscles and tendons that are brought into play to maintain balance. For best results start doing them *before* poor posture habits have had time to form.

FOOT EXERCISES

Your feet are the natural foundation for a good standing and walking posture. So take good care of them. During pregnancy, when your feet have to bear more than their usual load, they need all the help you can give them with good shoes, exercise, rest, and massage to prevent them from weakening under the unaccustomed strain. All it takes to keep your feet in good condition is some daily exercise and a conscious effort to stand and walk correctly: your toes flexed to secure a good grip on the ground (or intervening shoes), your soles arched, and your weight resting on the balls, outer borders, and heels of your feet.

The following are a few of the many simple but effective exercises for strengthening the muscles and tendons of the feet. Unlike other posture exercises foot exercises should be done throughout your entire pregnancy. You can do them standing (while brushing your teeth, washing the dishes, etc.) or sitting (while working at your desk or watching TV, etc.) so suit them to your day and do them regularly.

Tiptoe bends

Starting position:

Sit or stand (preferably barefoot) with feet side by side. For better balance in a standing position, hold on to a stable piece of furniture with one hand the first few times.

Movements:

1. Lift the heel of your right foot off the floor and go up on your toes as illustrated in Figure 2.2a. Hold for a count of 3.
2. Then go up on your tiptoes and hold for another count of 3 (Figure 2-2b).
3. Return foot into bent position, as in step 1, and then lower heel to floor as at the start.
4. Repeat 3–5 times with each foot.

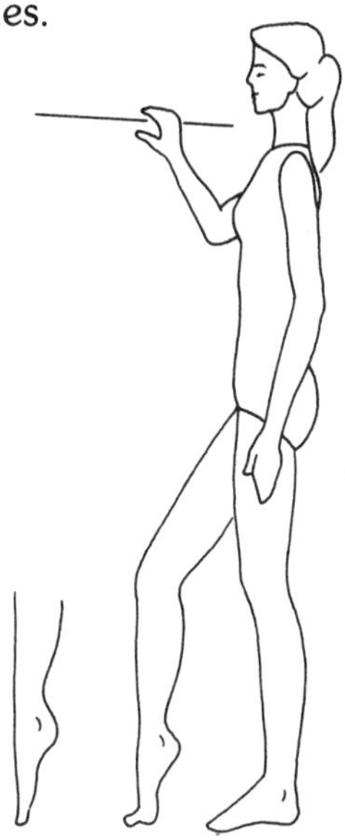

The caterpillar crawl

Starting position:
Same as for tiptoe bends.

Fig. 2-2B

Movements:

1. Starting with your right foot, firmly grip floor with bent toes, arching soles, and drawing heels up nearer to toes.
2. Then stretch toes out, keeping heels on the floor.
3. Continue to bend, grip, and stretch toes, inching foot forward along the floor in tiny caterpillar-like steps as far as is comfortable.
4. Retract your steps and return to start by reversing the movements of your toes.
5. Repeat with left foot.

Fig. 2-2A

Fig. 2-3

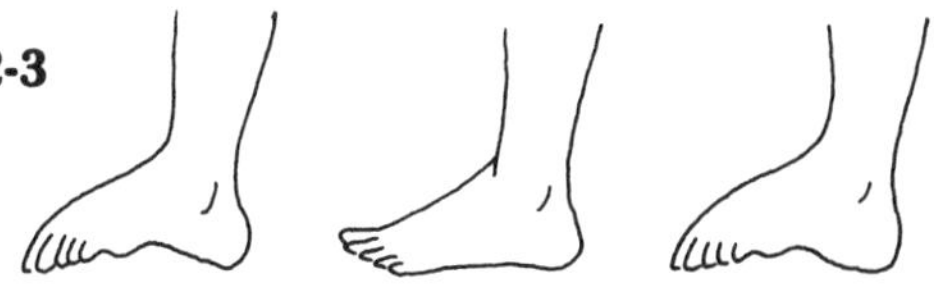

Pigeon-toed side-stands

Starting position:
Stand pigeon-toed with feet comfortably apart.

Movements:
Bend knees outward and curl toes in to stand on the outer borders of your feet (Figure 2-4). Repeat rhythmically 8-10 times.

To do this exercise while sitting, start with your legs together and proceed as follows:
1. Point toes inward (pigeon-toed fashion), sliding heels slightly out at the sides.
2. Curl toes in, bringing arches up and lowering outer borders of feet to floor as in Figure 2-5. Repeat 8-10 times.

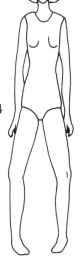

Fig. 2-4

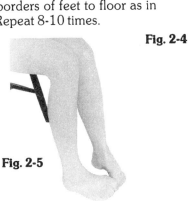

Fig. 2-5

End all footwork by shaking your feet vigorously, one at a time.

PELVIC-TILTING EXERCISES

When you keep your pelvis tilted up at just the right angle your baby is balanced securely inside the bony pelvic basin and your lower back and abdominal muscles are spared. To help you keep your pelvis tilted properly, in spite of the increased weight of your heavily laden pelvis and the forces of gravity, practice pelvic tilting often—every day, from your fourth month on. Besides improving your posture, and strengthening the muscles of your pelvic floor, rhythmically tilting your pelvis up and down helps firm your bottom and flatten your tummy. Once you've got the knack of it, you can practice almost anywhere, any time, whether sitting at a desk, standing in the kitchen, or waxing the floor on your hands and knees.

The leaning-back pelvic rock

Starting position:
Keeping back straight, neck well stretched, and head erect, sit back and lean on your hands, with palms flat on the floor behind you for support, fingers pointing in toward you. Bend and spread knees comfortably wide apart so that soles of feet touch.

Movements:
1. Inhale and working from below the waist thrust pelvis forward, tilting it down and relaxing buttocks, abdominal muscles, and pelvic floor muscles (Figure 2-6a). (To check if your pelvic floor muscles are relaxed, ask yourself if you could possibly relieve your bladder in this position.)
2. Exhale and tilt pelvis up, drawing tummy firmly in and tightening buttocks and pelvic floor muscles, as for bladder control (Figure 2-6b). Hold until you feel the need to inhale.
3. Repeat 6-8 times, keeping the movements rhythmic.

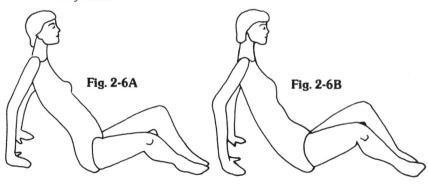

Fig. 2-6A   Fig. 2-6B

Now that you know how to do the pelvic rock sitting down, you're ready to practice standing on your own two feet. Just fold your arms in front at shoulder level (to help keep your upper body still), and work your pelvis independently of your torso, rocking it rhythmically back and forth, as if you were dancing to the beat of some exotic music. (Better still, do it to music.)

From here on whenever you do Program A, you can practice pelvic tilting either sitting or standing, whichever way suits you best.

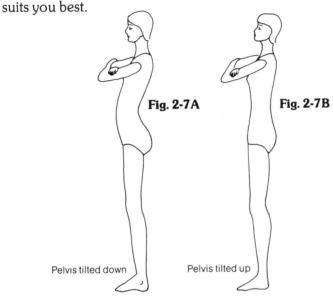

Fig. 2-7A   **Fig. 2-7B**

Pelvis tilted down   Pelvis tilted up

SPINE-S-T-R-E-T-C-H-I-N-G EXERCISES

Even if you manage to keep your pelvis tilted up at just the right angle and your feet well arched and firmly planted, you could spoil it all by letting your head and shoulders droop to look down at your feet. Don't! Think "tall" instead. Make it a point to carry yourself with your spine stretched from the tip of your tailbone to the base of your skull and your head balanced lightly at the very top, perfectly aligned with your neck and the rest of your spine.

The following exercises are designed to help you do just that.

The lying-down spine stretch

Starting position:

Lie flat on your back on the floor, body relaxed, arms naturally along sides, palms down, knees bent and drawn up at a 45-degree angle, together or slightly apart, with feet straight and soles flat on the floor.

Movements:

1. On an exhale, push the floor steadily away with the soles of your feet, without actually letting them slide forward; press small of back to floor, pull tummy in and tuck seat under, stretching spine along the floor so that neck "grows" longer and chin sinks slightly to chest.

2. Keeping spine stretched with small of back pressed to floor, bend right ankle back and slowly stretch right leg out as you exhale, gliding heel carefully forward along floor, as far as you can reach *without* lifting small of back off the floor (Figure 2-8).

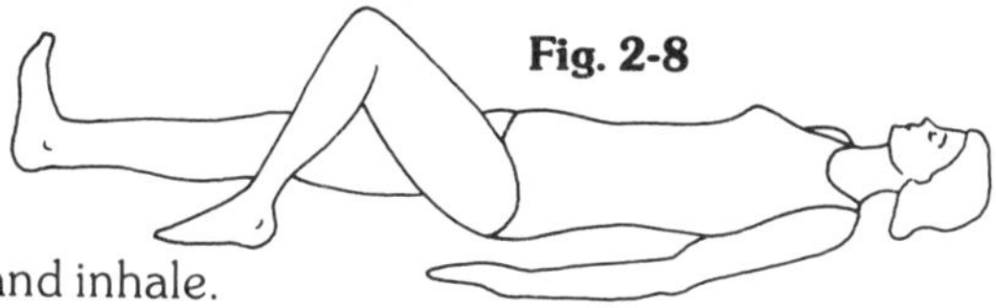

Fig. 2-8

3. Hold for a moment and inhale.

4. With your next breath out, slowly return right leg to starting position, carefully gliding heel back up along the floor while keeping small of back still pressed down. Don't lift your heel off the floor and don't point toes!

5. Once knee is drawn up at a 45-degree angle, inhale and set foot back down flat on the floor.

6. Alternating legs, do 3 times with each leg.

7. Now do it once with both legs, stretching first one and then the other (never both at once!) out along the floor as you exhale, with ankles bent and small of back pressed down throughout. When both legs are extended, hold and inhale. Then exhale

and slowly draw one leg after the other, backward along the floor to starting position, as in steps 4 and 5. Go slowly and easily. Remember this exercise is to help you develop a sense of posture as well as to improve muscle tone and spine flexibility.

8. Repeat 2 times and don't worry if at first you can't keep your knees straight when your legs are extended along the floor. More important is keeping the small of your back pressed to the floor. With practice you should be able to do both.

Now relax and get the "kinks" out of your spine by doing the following limbering-up exercise for easing tension and strain all along the spinal column.

Spine swinging

Starting position:
Lie on back with body relaxed, eyes closed, arms naturally along sides, hands open, knees bent and slightly parted, feet straight, and soles flat on the floor.

Movements:
1. Exhale and push steadily against the floor with the soles of your feet, bringing your spine to swing gently upward from the base, vertebra after vertebra, in a smooth, snaky motion. Don't force it! Go slowly and easily, working only with your feet and letting your spine take care of itself. The small of your back will press into the floor and your neck will arch somewhat, so that the head rolls slightly back and chin juts out. This movement usually takes some time and concentration to achieve.

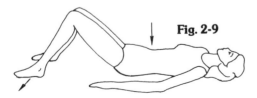

Fig. 2-9

2. Inhale and gently grip the floor with the soles of your feet to pull your body slightly downward (toward your feet), bringing spine to swing back into its natural curvatures at waist and neck levels. When done correctly, the head rolls slightly forward into starting position, with chin tucked in.

3 Using your feet for leverage, repeat steps 1 and 2 in a continuous, smooth motion, bringing the spine to swing gently back and forth for as long as you please.

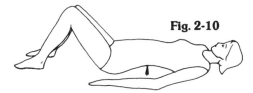

Fig. 2-10

Tip: *To help you experience the free-flowing motion of the spine, solicit the help of the father-to-be (or some other good friend). While you remain passive, resting in the described starting position, have your helper place his hands just above your knees and then gently pull them forward towards himself. (Feel how this slight movement sets your vertebrae into motion?) Then have him place his hand just below your knees and push them gently back, away from himself. (Feel the upward, wave-like motion of your spine?) Repeat the back and forth movements several times, in a smooth, continuous motion.*

Standing back-to-wall spine stretch

Starting position:
Stand "tall" with back to wall and feet about 6 inches away, straight and slightly apart. Let arms hang naturally at the sides.

Tip: *Close your eyes to intensify your sense of physical awareness.*

Movements:

1. On an inhale, "collapse" and "fold up" at the waist, letting lower back round out as shoulders slump forward and head rolls back along the wall (Figure 2-11a). Neck arches and chin juts out. When this is done correctly, your knees bend slightly and your pelvis is drawn up toward your ribs. (Check this by placing your hands on your hip bones to see if they turn up.)

2. While exhaling, push away from the floor with your feet to pull yourself up to a tall, upright position, straightening knees, drawing the tummy in, and stretching your spine from top to bottom. The small of the back eases off the wall (arching naturally) and neck "grows" longer, bringing head up along the wall to look straight ahead. (See Figure 2-11b.) Check whether buttocks, shoulder blades, and back of head are still in contact with the wall, with crown pointing up to ceiling. If not, then something is wrong with your posture.

3. Repeat 3-4 times, moving in a smooth, free-flowing rhythm.

Back-to-wall spinal roll

Starting position:
Stand "tall" with back to wall, arms hanging naturally along sides, knees slightly flexed, feet straight, somewhat parted and about 6 inches away from the wall. Close your eyes to enhance physical awareness.

Movements:

1. On an exhale, drop head and slowly "fall" forward, letting head, arms and torso dangle loosely like a rag doll (Figures 2-12a, b, c). (Buttocks must remain in contact with the wall!) Relax and inhale.

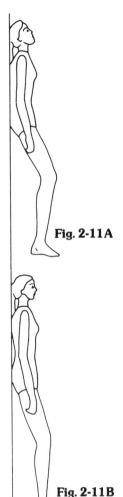

Fig. 2-11A

Fig. 2-11B

2. Then exhale; pull tummy in, flex knees slightly, and using feet for leverage, push off from the floor and slowly pull yourself up to a standing position, one vertebra at a time, starting at the base of the spine and pressing first the "tail" (coccyx), small of back, and then upper back, firmly to wall, with head still hanging down, heavy with the drag of gravity (Figure 2-12d).
3. Slowly straighten the top seven cervical vertebrae as you inhale, pulling bowed head upright.
4. Pause a moment at the top before opening your eyes.
5. Repeat 1–2 times, always taking a short rest before starting again.

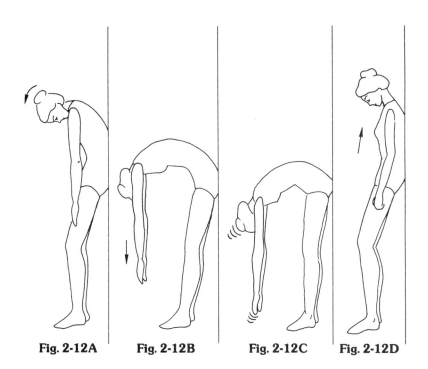

Fig. 2-12A   Fig. 2-12B   Fig. 2-12C   Fig. 2-12D

The free-standing spinal roll

Once you have mastered the back-to-wall spinal roll, try the exercise standing free, with feet shoulder-width apart and firmly planted. To help you do it just right, study the following illustrations.

Going down

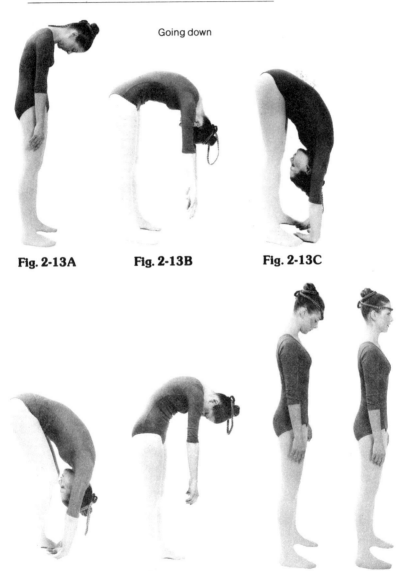

Fig. 2-13A   Fig. 2-13B   Fig. 2-13C

Fig. 2-13D   Fig. 2-13E   Fig. 2-13F   Fig. 2-13G

EXERCISES FOR BALANCE AND POISE

The final ingredient essential to your posture is a sense of balance and poise—that very special way of carrying yourself with ease and a certain self-possessed manner, with every part of your body loosely in tow.

The following exercises will help you acquire this quality.

Puppet-on-a-string

Starting position:
Stand "tall" with shoulders relaxed (back and down), knees loose, feet straight, side by side, and soles firmly planted.

Movements:

1. Close your eyes; tighten seat and back of thigh muscles, press hands against sides of thighs (in stiff military fashion), and imagine yourself to be a wooden puppet suspended at the crown by a string attached to the ceiling and fixed firmly to the floor at the soles of your feet.

2. Still thinking "puppet-on-a-string," flex your toes to get a good grip on the floor and keep them firmly planted, and tilt torso stiffly forward, without losing your balance. Then tilt torso backward. Teeter to and fro several times before returning to center.

3. Maintaining your balance and contact with both the ceiling above and the floor below, lean stiffly to one side and then to the other. Keep on swaying slowly from side to side and then gradually begin rotating head and torso in small, carefully measured circles, as if you were drawing circles on the ceiling with the top of your head (Figure 2-14). Stop after 3-4 rounds and circle in the opposite direction 3-4 times.

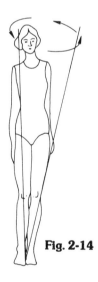

Fig. 2-14

4. End by first slowing down and then returning to center. Pause briefly, then open your eyes to look straight ahead. Check your posture. If you did this exercise correctly, it will be exactly as it was in the starting position.

The warming-up walk

Starting position:

With feet slightly apart, stand erect but not stiff (preferably in front of a full-length mirror) and make a conscious effort to do all of the following:

1. Flex toes to get a good grip on the floor (or intervening shoes) with your weight falling evenly on the balls, outer borders, and heels of your feet. (When this is done correctly, feet are arched and somewhat smaller.)

2. Relax knees. (To help loosen them, flex knees a little and bounce lightly a few times.)

3. Lightly tense seat muscles, pinching buttocks slightly together.

4. Tilt pelvis up, "cradling" the baby safely within the pelvic basin and tucking seat under.

5. Pull tummy in.

6. Lift rib cage and "grow" taller and slimmer between hips and lower ribs *without* raising shoulders in stiff military fashion. (Check to see if shoulders and arms are relaxed by gently swinging them to and fro.)

7. Stretch neck, making it longer and adding to the distance between shoulders and ears.

8. Look straight ahead and hold head upright with chin in and top of head pointing up at the ceiling, as illustrated in Figure 2-15a.

9. Use your imagination—it can work wonders for your posture. To help keep spine (including neck) and head aligned, pretend that your head is a balloon, attached to your spine instead of to a string, and let it pull your body up as tall as it will go (Figure 2-15b). Or, if that doesn't work, try thinking of yourself as a puppet being

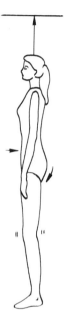

Fig. 2-15A

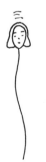

Fig. 2-15B

pulled up toward the ceiling by a string attached at the top of your head (Figure 2-15c). Keeping either thought in mind, go from standing to walking by first tilting yourself slightly forward to shift the line of gravity of your body forward. Then lift and swing one leg to the front, bending it at the knee, while the other leg supports your inclined body and provides the necessary push-off.

With shoulders back and relaxed, and arms hanging down at the sides, look straight ahead and let your body float along, propelled forward by your legs and pulled up tall by your head, your spine stretched from top to tail.

Walk with light, springy steps and a bounce of vitality as you smoothly swing one leg forward and push off with the other, bending your knees and working thighs and toes as you go. Start slowly and work up to a lively, brisk pace continuing for 1-2 minutes before gradually decreasing your speed at the end.

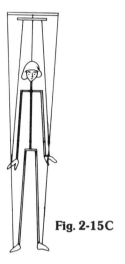

Fig. 2-15C

Add some variety and spice to your walk by taking a few steps up on your toes or on your heels as you move along. Try such simple combinations as: step-step-toe-toe-heel-heel, or heel-toe-heel-toe, keeping your movements rhythmic and consciously maintaining your balance and posture throughout. (Pretend you're carrying a jug of water on your head.) Some other good variations are walking on the outer borders of your feet (Figure 2-16c) and walking with your feet firmly arched and toes curled in (Figure 2-16d).

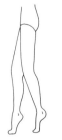
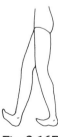
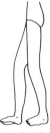
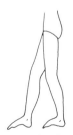

Fig. 2-16A   Fig. 2-16B   Fig. 2-16C   Fig. 2-16D

Just for fun try a few rhythmic kickbacks as well. Bend right leg at the knee and kick heel back up and across to left buttock (Figure 2-17). Then swing right leg forward to step ahead. Alternating legs, do kick-step-kick for several paces, keeping all movements rhythmic and increasing your tempo as you go.

Tip: *This vigorous 1- to 2-minute "walk" around the room is an excellent way to warm up at the start of any exercise session.*

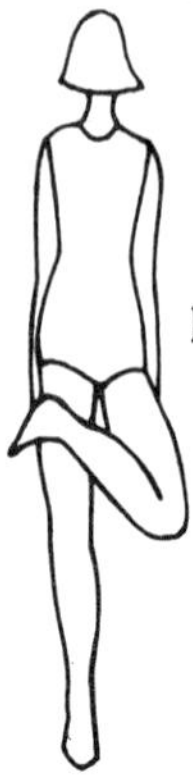

Fig. 2-17

FIRMING AND TONING

Now that you've stirred up your circulation and sent a good flow of blood to your muscles and tendons, your body is warm and loose, ready to be toned and firmed from head to toe. So turn on the music and try the following invigorating exercises.

The heel-toe-roll

For ankles, calves, and for improving circulation in legs.

Starting position:
Stand "tall," one leg stretched out and placed in front of the other, with toes pointing down and touching the floor (Figure 2-18a). If necessary, hold on to something stable with one hand for better balance.

Movements:
1. Keeping stretched leg stiff with knees straight, flex ankle back, pointing toes up and touch heel to floor (Figure 2-18b).
2. Then stretch ankle, lifting heel off floor and touch toes to floor again.

3. Continue doing heel-toe, heel-toe for a slow count of 10.
4. Then still keeping knee straight, raise your extended foot slightly off the floor and roll it around clockwise, in a wide arc (Figure 2-18c), 3-5 times, before tapping the floor once with your big toe. Reverse the movements, rolling foot around in the opposite direction 3-5 times before tapping big toe to floor.

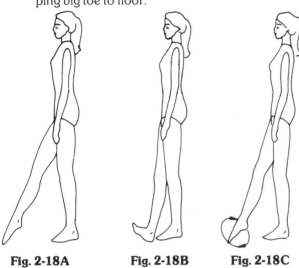

Fig. 2-18A   **Fig. 2-18B**   **Fig. 2-18C**

5. Reverse position of legs and repeat steps 1 through 4 with other leg.
6. Follow up by shaking both legs vigorously, one at a time, to de-tense them.

One-legged knee bends
For thighs, buttocks, and balance.

Starting position:
Standing tall with feet together.

Movements:
1. On an inhale slide right foot forward (Figure 2-19a) and lift arms gracefully out at the sides for balance.

2. Keeping upper body erect, exhale; bend both knees, and lower yourself smoothly and easily on your left knee, which should be directly under your hip (Figure 2-19b). Go down as far as you can reach and bounce 3 times.
3. Breathing naturally, rise slowly, using only "thigh power."
4. Without stopping, slide your left leg smoothly forward and go down gracefully on your right knee, repeating the one-legged knee bend in a reversed position.

    Do 4-6 knee bends on alternate sides.

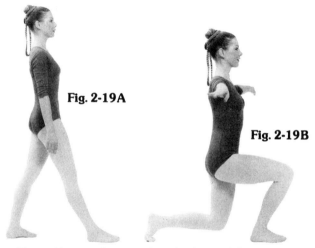

Fig. 2-19A

Fig. 2-19B

Note: *Always take care that the lowered knee and thigh are directly in line with hip and shoulder on the same side.*

Bent-knee swings

For inner thighs and for improving circulation in the external iliac veins running through the groins.

Starting position:

Stand "tall," feet together, arms extended loosely at the sides with one hand holding on to some firm, stationary piece of furniture.

Movements:

1. On an exhale lift right knee up in front with toes pointed down; touch toes lightly to left kneecap to help you maintain your balance (Figure 2-20a).
2. Inhale and swing raised knee sideways to the right, reaching as far as it can go (Figure 2-20b).
3. Exhale and swing raised knee around to the left, crossing it over left thigh (Figure 2-20c).

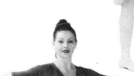

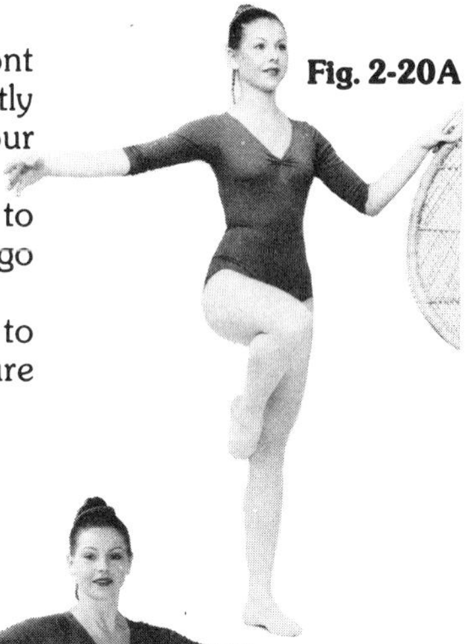

Fig. 2-20A

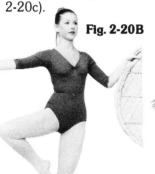

Fig. 2-20B

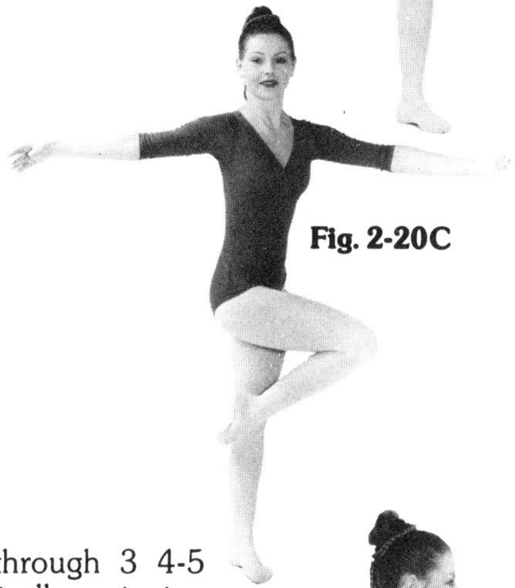

Fig. 2-20C

4. Repeat movements 1 through 3 4-5 times, nonstop, rhythmically swinging bent knee back and forth and letting your breathing take care of itself.
5. Repeat with your other leg.

The kick-up

For firming upper thigh muscles.

Starting position:

Same as for bent-knee swings.

Movements:

1. Exhale as you slowly bend and lift knee of one leg up high with toes pointing down (Figure 2-21a).

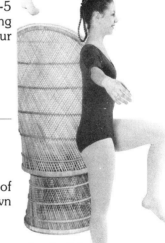

Fig. 2-21A

2. Inhale and quickly kick up calf of raised leg, extending the entire leg in mid-air and tensing it from toe to top of thigh (Figure 2-21b). Hold a moment.
3. Then exhale and abruptly drop calf, letting it hang down limply from the joint while keeping thigh up in front.
4. Breathing naturally, continue to alternately kick and drop the calf of your raised leg, 2-3 more times; end by giving one last kick with your raised leg to help it reach higher before letting it drop limply to the floor.
5. Repeat with other leg.
6. Follow up by shaking both legs vigorously, one at a time, to de-tense them.

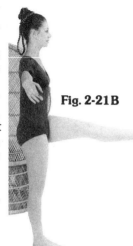

Fig. 2-21B

The leg twister
For hips, buttocks, thighs, waist, and spine flexibility.

Starting position:
The same as for bent-knee swings.

Breathing instructions:
Start on an exhale and continue to breathe naturally as you go.

Movements:
1. Slowly bend and raise right knee, bringing it up as high as it can go, with toes pointing down.
2. Swing it around to your right side.
3. Kick right calf up, extending leg at the side, in line with hip or as high as it can reach, keeping knee perfectly straight, parallel to ceiling and toes pointed (Figure 2-22a).
4. Leaning torso, but not head, slightly to the left for balance and holding on with your left hand to a wall, or some piece of

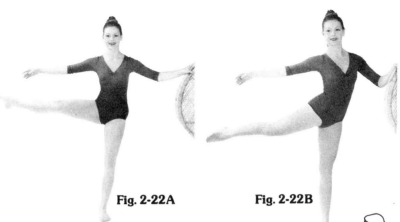

Fig. 2-22A   Fig. 2-22B

furniture, turn right kneecap down to face
floor, twisting right leg and turning right
hip to the limit (Figure 2-22b).

5. Then, working from the hip, untwist leg
and turn kneecap back up to face ceiling.
Rhythmically twist and untwist extended
leg 3-4 times, before slowly lowering it to
the floor.

6. Now de-tense by alternately swinging
your legs lazily back and forth several
times, keeping your moving knee loose
so that it bends naturally as it comes up in
front. (See Figure 2-22c.)

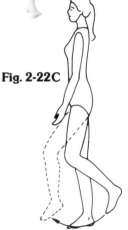

Fig. 2-22C

The stilted walk

*A standing hip-shrugging exercise for your
waist muscles and for loosening up the sacroiliac joints in the lower back.*

Breathing instructions:
Shrug on an exhale, stretch on an inhale.

Starting position:
Stand erect with legs and arms stiff, keeping
arms close to sides, in strict military fashion,

with wrists bent so that palms face the floor. Knees should be blocked back hard and feet somewhat apart, turned slightly inward (pigeon-toed).

Movements:
1. Keeping head as still as possible and legs very stiff with ankles flexed and feet turned slightly inward, "shrug" first one hip and then the other, "stepping" stiffly in place as if standing on stilts. (See Figure 2-23.) Don't swing your hips!
2. Do 8-12 shrugs, alternating hips.
3. Then, breathing naturally, try taking about 6 "stilted" steps forward and then a few steps back, "walking" stiffly and keeping your pace rhythmic.

Tip: *Keep legs very stiff throughout this exercise.*

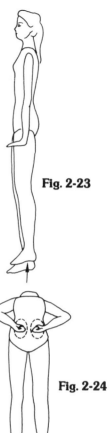

Fig. 2-23

4. Now clench hands to make fists, bend head and torso forward and finish off by massaging your posterior iliac spine (just beneath the two skin "dimples" of your back) with the flat, inner sides of your fists, where thumb and index finger meet. See Figure 2-24.

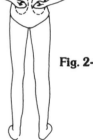

Fig. 2-24

The forward spinal-bend
For the lumbar vertebrae and the abdominal muscles.

Starting position:
Stand erect with legs slightly apart and arms extended loosely at the sides.

Movements:
1. Exhale and in a smooth, continuous motion tilt pelvis up (tucking seat under and pulling tummy in) and gracefully bend and lift right knee up high, with toes of raised foot pointing down, while simultaneously bending your left knee out at

the side, rounding your back to bring torso slightly forward and slowly swinging arms forward to join hands lightly in front of raised knee (Figure 2-25).

2. Then inhale and slowly return to starting position.
3. Alternating legs, do 3 times with each leg.

The backward arm lift
For shoulders, bust and chest expansion.

Starting positions:
Stand "tall," legs spread comfortably apart, arms stretched out behind you and fingers interlaced with palms facing up to ceiling.

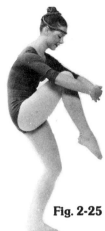

Fig. 2-25

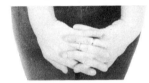

Fig. 2-26A

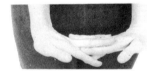

Fig. 2-26B

Fig. 2-26C

Movements:
1. Twist hands around, turn palms toward back (Figure 2-26a); then twist hands down to floor, so that thumbs separate (Figure 2-26b).
2. Inhale; bend forward from the waist while lifting arms up high behind you and roll head back to look straight ahead (Figure 2-26c). Hold until your lungs are filled.
3. Exhale and return to starting position.
4. Repeat twice.

The pectoral press

For bust.

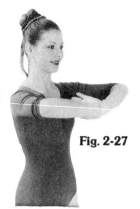

Fig. 2-27

Starting position:
Stand "tall," feet spread comfortably apart and palms of hands together in front of chest with fingers pointing in (Figure 2-27).

Movements:
1. Exhale and press hands together. Press harder and harder and harder!
2. Relax and inhale.
3. Repeat 3 times.

The crisscross arm stretch

For the arms.

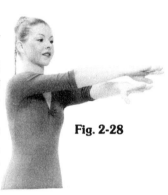

Fig. 2-28

Starting position:
Stand erect with feet comfortably apart and arms stretched out straight in front at shoulder level, with hands crossed one over the other.

Movements:
1. Keeping hands close and arms stiff, cross and crisscross your hands, 10-12 times, without letting them touch (Figure 2-28). Increase your tempo as you go.
2. Relax and shake arms out to de-tense.
3. Repeat once.

The roll-around

For getting out the kinks in your neck.

Starting position:
Stand "tall," with feet comfortably apart, arms hanging down limply at the sides, and eyes closed to enhance your sense of physical awareness and relaxation.

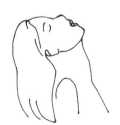

Fig. 2-29A

Movements:
1. Drop head forward, letting it hang down limply. Then straighten the top seven vertebrae in the neck to pull head up to its erect standing position (Figure 2-29a).
2. Drop head back, letting lips part naturally. Then slowly return to upright position.

3. Drop head to the right. Then slowly pull it back up again to center. Do the same on the left side (Figure 2-29b).

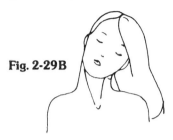

Fig. 2-29B

4. Follow up by dropping head forward and letting it loll lazily around several times, first in one direction and then in the other. Ignore any crackling and keep on going until all (or almost all) the kinks are out.
5. End by pulling head back up to starting position and then opening your eyes to look straight ahead.

SQUATTING

The wobbly, disjointed feeling typical of late pregnancy is caused by the normal loosening-up effect of pregnancy hormones on the pelvic joints and their connecting ligaments. Normally the three pelvic joints (two in the back and one in the front) are constructed so that very little motion is possible. But during pregnancy they actually grow farther apart, in order to widen the birth canal and enable the baby to pass through the bony pelvis. To further this natural loosening-up process and to make spreading your thighs during delivery more comfortable, squatting during pregnancy is a must.

Fortunately, squatting takes only a few seconds of your time and can be done almost anywhere, holding on to anything solid and stable of reasonable height, such as the kitchen sink, two doorknobs, a bathtub, a desk, or even a husband.

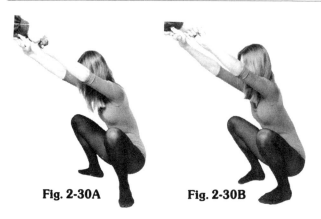

Fig. 2-30A   Fig. 2-30B

In Figure 2-30a, the feet are turned slightly outward, causing arches to be flattened to floor; this position is to be avoided. In Figure 2-30b, however, the feet are turned somewhat inward at the start so that the arches are protected. As you can see, by squatting with your feet turned slightly inward (pigeon-toed fashion) you can stretch your thigh muscles, widen your pelvis, and strengthen your arches all at once.

The holding-on squat

Starting position:
With feet spread hip-width apart, stand arm's distance away from an open door (sink, etc.) and grasp the doorknobs on either side (or the front of the sink, etc.).

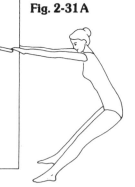

Fig. 2-31 A

Movements
1. Pull away from the door, straightening elbows and knees and pushing bottom out as far back as it will go, bringing yourself to bend forward at the waist (Figure 2-31 a).

2. When you've gone as far back as you can go, bend knees out at the side and squat down slowly, keeping heels flat on the floor (Figure 2-31b). Relax except for your hands, and bounce 3-5 times (Figure 2-31c).
3. Still holding on tightly to doorknobs, push the floor away with your feet and pull yourself away from the door by slowly straightening knees and sweeping bottom up and out behind you as far as it can reach, so that you naturally bend forward at the waist.
4. Then tug on the doorknobs and bend elbows out at the sides to bring yourself up to starting position.
5. Repeat 2-3 times.

Note: *After you can do this exercise easily, practice squatting without holding on. Then make it a habit always to squat down instead of bending forward from the waist whenever you have to reach down to floor level to pick something up or open a drawer, etc. Proper position is illustrated in Figure 2-32.*

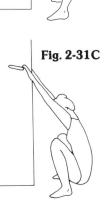

Fig. 2-31B

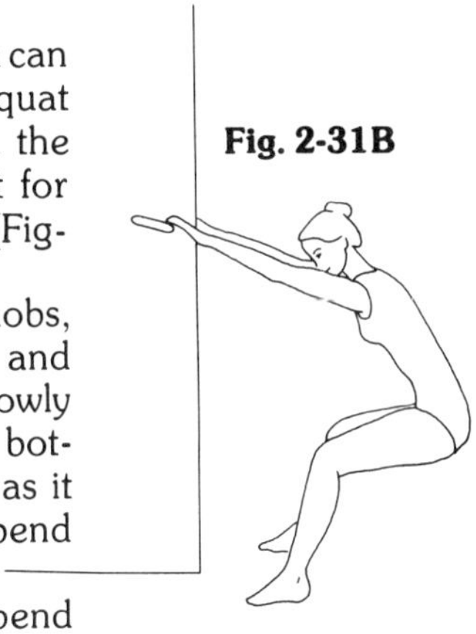

Fig. 2-31C

Fig. 2-32

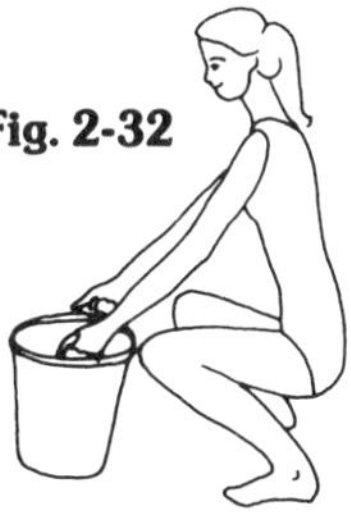

To complete your workout for the day and help pump the old blood out of your legs and pelvic veins, lie down on your back on the floor and do some spine-rolling, as described on page 92.

Then roll over and rest on your side with elbows and knees flexed. Close your eyes and relax, breathing naturally for as long as you please. When you're ready rise slowly in stages and open your eyes.

Chapter Three

PROGRAM B

PROTECTING THE PECTORALS

For pregnant bosoms, fighting the forces of gravity can be a losing battle without the support of a well-fitted bra and some daily exercise. Done regularly, throughout your entire pregnancy, the few simple exercises in this section can help you retain the pre-pregnant contours of your breasts and prevent your back from aching and your shoulders from drooping under the extra weight of your breasts. By improving circulation, they also help get a good flow of blood to the glandular and supportive tissues, which in turn improves your chances of adequate milk production later on.

The bosom bounce

Breathing instructions:
Always inhale deeply and then hold your breath as you bounce bosom rhythmically up and down 10 times.

Starting position:
Sit or stand "tall," with arms held up at shoulder level, bent at the elbows.

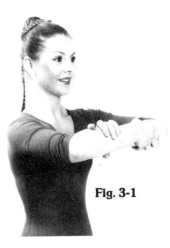

Movements:
1. Grasp arms above wrist, and holding on very tightly, forcefully push back the skin without letting hands slide up arms (Figure 3-1).
2. Relax and repeat rhythmically 10 times.
3. Lift arms in front of your nose and do 10 more bosom bounces at this higher level.

Fig. 3-1

Note: *If you watch yourself in a mirror, you should be able to see your bosom bouncing with each push.*

/59

Elbow push-backs

Breathing instructions:
Start on an exhale and continue to breathe naturally.

Starting position:
Sit near the edge of your chair or bed, leaning forward, with hands on shoulders and elbows bent out at the sides. Tilt torso forward with back straight, aligned with neck and head (Figure 3-2a).

Movements:
1. Keeping back straight, twist torso to the right to look at right elbow (Figure 3-2b).
2. Then push right elbow back, giving 2-3 little thrusts to help you reach farther.
3. Twist torso to the left and push left elbow back (Figure 3-2c) giving 2-3 little thrusts.
4. Alternating sides, do 2-3 times on each side.

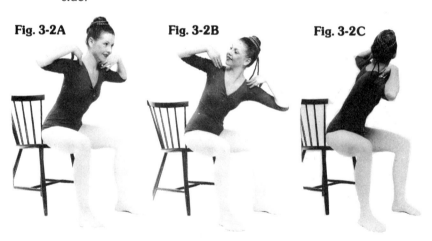

Fig. 3-2A   Fig. 3-2B   Fig. 3-2C

Elbow circling

Breathing instructions:
For steps 1 and 2 inhale as elbows "inscribe" the upper half of the circle and chest naturally expands, exhale as it completes the lower

half of the circle. For steps 3 and 4 the trick is to remember to keep on breathing, not to hold in your breath.

Starting position:
Same as for elbow push-backs.

Movements:
1. Keeping back straight and tilted forward, slowly swing bent elbows around in a big wide circle, moving them forward (Figure 3-3a); up high, brushing ears with hands (Figure 3-3b); back (Figure 3-3c) and down behind you (Figure 3-3d). Complete 3 non-stop circles.

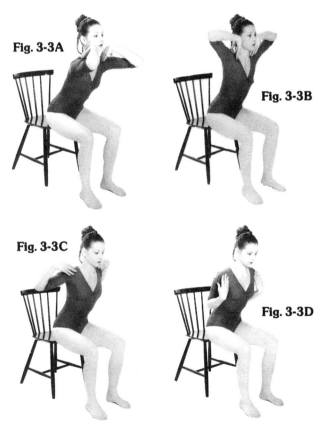

Fig. 3-3A

Fig. 3-3B

Fig. 3-3C

Fig. 3-3D

2. Reversing the movements, do 3 more times, swinging elbows backward (Figure 3-3c), up, around to the front, and back down to starting position (Figure 3-3d).
3. Do a few more elbow-circles, swinging both arms in opposite directions, so that one circles backward while the other circles forward. Gradually increase speed and vigor as you go.
4. Then abruptly reverse directions (i.e., the elbow that went forward now goes backward and vice versa) and swing your elbows around quickly and vigorously several times more.
5. Stop and pause to catch your breath. Breathing should be easier and deeper.

Tip: *Brush sides of chest with arms as you bring elbows forward.*

Arm-twist
For arms, shoulders, and neck.

Starting position:
Sit or stand "tall," arms stretched out straight at the sides with palm of left hand facing down to the floor and palm of right hand facing up toward the ceiling.

Breathing instructions:
Start each movement on an inhale and continue to breathe slowly and deeply as you go.

Movements:
1. Keeping both arms stiff, twist right hand all the way around, turning palm forward, down, backward, and up—so that right shoulder rolls forward—and turn your head gracefully to look over your hunched shoulder at your twisting hand (Figure 3-4a).
2. Reverse the movements, slowly unwinding the twisted hand and arm while returning shoulder and head to starting position.

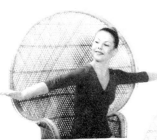

Fig. 3-4A

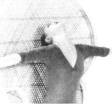

Fig. 3-4B

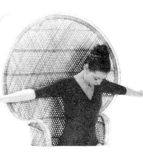

3. Repeat 2-3 times with your right arm, always moving your working arm in a slow, sensuous motion and turning your head gracefully to look at your hunched shoulder.

Fig. 3-4C

4. Then reverse positions of hands (right hand facing down and left facing up) and do 3-4 more complete twists with your left arm.

5. Now turn palms of both hands up and do it 6 more times with both arms simultaneously, letting head roll gently back with each double twist and curling it slowly forward to chest as arms "unwind." (Figures 3-4b and 3-4c)

6. Follow up by bending elbows and shaking arms and hands vigorously to de-tense them.

CHECKING YOUR "UNDERCARRIAGE"

High on the list of pregnancy woes is damage to the pelvic-vaginal muscles. Yet all it takes to protect your "undercarriage" are a few, simple, easygoing exercises that take only seconds to do. Done regularly, throughout your entire pregnancy, you can improve muscle tone, control, and circulation in the pelvic floor and prevent the urinary stress incontinence (slight loss of bladder control upon such stress as coughing and sneezing) that annoys so many mothers.

The bottom bounce

Breathing instruction:
Start on an exhale and continue to breathe naturally.

Starting position:
Sit near the edge of a firm chair, with knees hip-width apart and feet flat on the floor. Keeping back very straight, perfectly aligned with neck and head, lean forward to rest hands lightly on thighs.

Movements:
1. Slowly tighten the muscles of the pelvic floor, contracting first the muscle fibers at the back (as if to check a bowel movement) and then those at the front (as for bladder control).
2. Maintaining the tension in your pelvic floor, quickly tighten your buttocks and feel yourself bouncing up. Squeeze hard to hold your "bounce" for a moment.
3. Then slowly relax buttocks and pelvic floor, letting bottom flatten against the chair.
4. Repeat twice.
5. Then for an extra firming effect, try bouncing quickly up and down, 3-5 times, rhythmically contracting and releasing both pelvic floor and seat muscles at once.

The ladylike lift

Breathing instruction:
Start on an exhale and continue to breathe naturally.

Starting position:
Same as for the bottom bounce. You can also do it sitting tailor fashion on the floor or

standing, although you won't be able to feel the "bounce."

Movements:

1. On an exhale tighten buttocks and "bounce" up. Then, imagining your vagina to be an "elevator" or "lift," tighten and draw it up, taking the "lift" from ground level up to your navel on the "third floor."
2. Hold a moment.
3. Trying to maintain your bounce, slowly lower your lift from third floor to second ... from second to first ... and finally back down to ground level. Only after it touches bottom, relax buttocks, letting it sink back down and flatten.
4. Repeat 2 to 3 times, always taking care to tense and hold at each "floor" on your way down.

Note: *Don't get discouraged if at first your "lift" seems somewhat "out of order." Doing this exercise properly takes practice, but it can be done. So keep on trying.*

Stop-and-go exercises

Doing these stop-and-go exercises is probably the best way to train your pelvic-vaginal muscles and at the same time check whether your actions are effective.

1. Whenever you empty your bladder, make it a point to interrupt the flow in midstream 2 to 3 times by tightly tensing your urethra and vagina and then slowly relaxing them.
2. When moving your bowels, try to keep back the movement at least once by tightening and closing your anus.

Once you know how, you can practice these simple, subtle movements anytime, anywhere—while riding the subway, waiting for a bus or watching television—without being noticed.

GETTING DOWN ON ALL FOURS

Besides being an extremely comfortable and relaxing way to exercise during pregnancy, the on-all-fours position also helps relieve circulatory congestion in the pelvic area and backache in the sacro-lumbar region. Kneeling on hands and knees automatically shifts the weight of the baby off the "little nerves" in your spine and gives your crowded inner organs a chance to fall back into place—suspended from the spine like clothes hanging on a line, instead of being crammed by the ever-growing, pregnant uterus. So make it a point to exercise, or at least rest, in the all-fours position for a minute or two every day.

THE BASIC ON-ALL-FOURS POSITION

Get down on your hands and knees as in Figure 3-5, with knees directly under hips, arms under shoulders and hands turned slightly inward. Keep tummy in, seat tucked under, and back straight, with head, neck, and spine aligned and face parallel to the floor. Feet may be together or apart, whichever suits you best.

Fig. 3-5

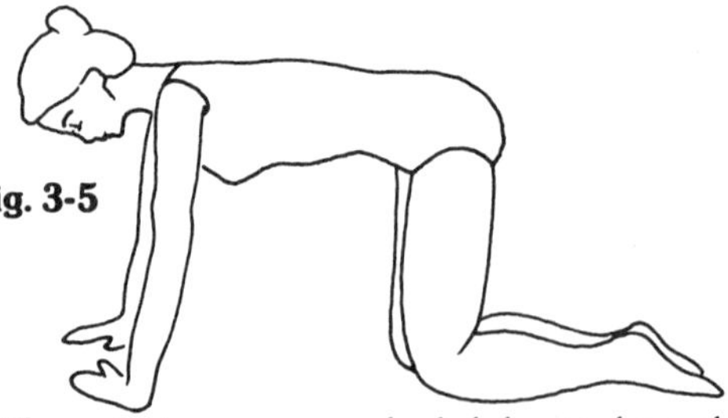

Important! *To protect your overworked abdominal muscles in this position, take special care not to let your back sag in the middle. Even when an exercise calls for arching the small of the back, don't overdo it by letting it cave in all the way.*

The pelvic rock on all fours

Starting position:
Basic on-all-fours position.

Movements:
1. Inhale and let small of back sag slightly, tilting pelvis down and relaxing seat and abdominal muscles. At the same time roll

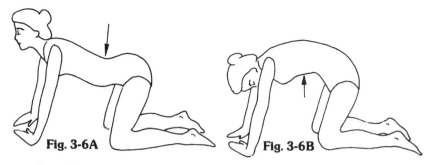

Fig. 3-6A

Fig. 3-6B

head back to look straight ahead. (See
Figure 3-6a.)

2. Exhale and simultaneously tighten buttocks, pelvic floor muscles, and lower
abdominal muscles, tucking seat snugly
under and pulling tummy firmly in toward
spine so that back (not shoulders!) is
humped up at waist level and head rolls
back down to look at floor. (See Figure
3-6b.) Make sure not to hunch shoulders
or hump up upper back!

3. Repeat 3-4 times.

The merry-go-round stretch

*Especially beneficial for the pectorals, the
neck, and for the prevention and relief of
backache.*

Starting position:
Sit back lightly on your heels, torso tilted
forward, back straight, arms stretched out
loosely in front, with palms flat on the floor
(Figure 3-7a).

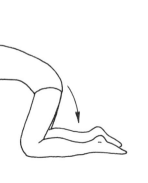

Fig. 3-7A

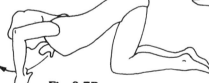

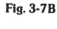

Fig. 3-7B

Fig. 3-7C

Movements:
1. While inhaling, slowly lower chest to floor, arching back, bending elbows outward, turning hands inward and rolling head back as you descend (Figure 3-7b).
2. Sweeping the floor with your bosom (as far as is comfortable), glide torso smoothly forward and then upward off the floor into a low, awkward, on-all-fours position, with head thrown back, small of back arched and elbows bent outward.
3. Then in one smooth continuous motion, exhale; hump back, straightening elbows and dropping head forward (Figure 3-7c) and . . .
4. . . . lower yourself, returning seat to heels and completing the circle.
5. Do the down-forward-up-and-around movement 3-5 times, moving in a smooth-flowing, circular motion. Then do it 3-5 more times, circling in reverse: up-around-down-and-back along the floor. In this direction, reverse the breathing pattern as well, inhaling on your way up and exhaling on your way down.

Leg-swinging spinal twist

For buttocks, waist and lower back.

Starting position:
Basic on-all-fours position, except that legs are together.

Movements:
1. Stretch right leg straight out behind you along the floor, with toes pointed, as in Figure 3-8a.

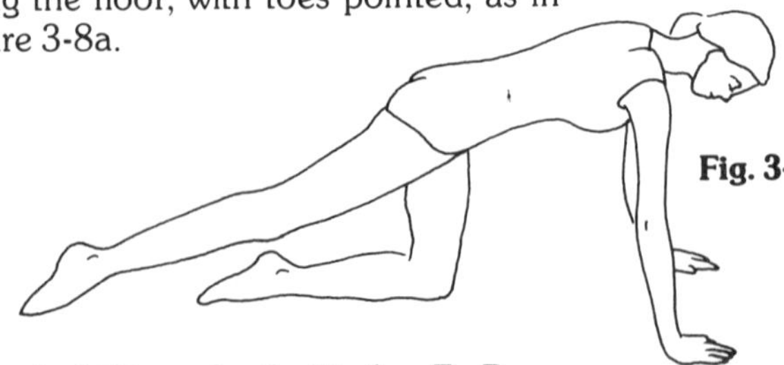

Fig. 3-8A

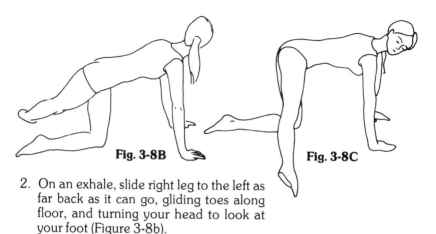

Fig. 3-8B

Fig. 3-8C

2. On an exhale, slide right leg to the left as far back as it can go, gliding toes along floor, and turning your head to look at your foot (Figure 3-8b).
3. Then inhale and swing right leg all the way around to the right, inscribing a half-circle on the floor with your toes and turning your head to look at your foot (Figure 3-8c).
4. Making sure to keep back straight and tummy in, do 10-12 nonstop back and forth swings with each leg, always touching toes of swinging leg to floor.

The arm-swinging torso-twist.

For spine flexibility, chest expansion, toning the oblique abdominal muscles and improving the circulation.

Starting position:
Basic all-fours position.

Movements:
1. While s-l-o-w-l-y exhaling through your mouth, swing right arm under left armpit and up toward the ceiling, twisting torso and head to look up at the pointed fingertips of your right hand (Figure 3-9a). Reach higher by giving 3 little rhythmic thrusts with your right arm while prolonging the exhalation by softly blowing through your mouth (*sssssss*...).

Fig. 3-9A

2. When all the air is expelled from your lungs, swing right arm back down, under and up to the right, turning torso and head to look up at your raised fingertips. Inhale with relish on your way up and *feel* the right side of your rib cage expanding.
3. Do 3 complete "swings" with your right arm; then rest a moment and repeat 3 more "swings" with your left arm.

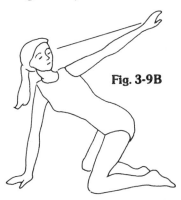

Fig. 3-9B

4. Follow with the shake down: Rise to a simple kneeling position, with your legs somewhat less apart than when kneeling on all fours, and shake hands and arms vigorously to de-tense them.

Now, since you're already in position for it, fold your arms in front at shoulder level, grasping elbows with hands, and do the torso tilt.

The torso tilt
A multipurpose exercise for thigh, seat, tummy, and upper back.

Breathing instructions:
Exhale as you lean back and inhale as you stretch forward.

Starting position:
See end of previous exercise.

Movements:

1. Keeping back very straight and seat tucked under, lean back as low as you can go without losing control of your straight back (Figure 3-10a). Bounce torso lightly 3 times to help lower your reach. (Feel the stretch in your thighs?)

2. Using only your thigh muscles, pull yourself back up to starting position.

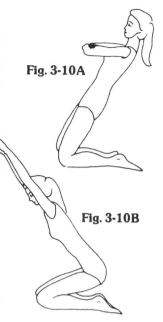

Fig. 3-10A

Fig. 3-10B

3. Then in one smooth, continuous motion, tilt torso forward, lower your bottom to about three inches off your heels and stretch arms out, bringing them together overhead* to form a straight line from hands to tailbone. Reach steadily forward with your outstretched arms, keeping back straight, seat tucked under, and tummy in (Figure 3-10b).

Tip: To help you keep arms, head, and spine aligned, keep upper arms close to ears and neck straight as you stretch forward.

4. Repeat 3-5 times.

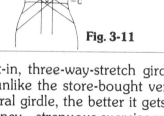

Fig. 3-11

TUMMY CONTROL

You were born with a built-in, three-way-stretch girdle of muscle (Figure 3-11), and unlike the store-bought version, the more you use your natural girdle, the better it gets. But don't *overdo* it during pregnancy—strenuous exercise may be too much for your already strained abdominal muscles. Remember that the more stretched out a muscle becomes, the less able it is to work effectively. It's like a rubber band: a gentle tensing and releasing action keeps it flexible, but stretch it too far and it's liable to snap. So if you want to be the

---

*Stretching both arms overhead is allowed in this case since torso is tilted forward and knees are bent.

woman with the flattest "tummy" on the maternity ward, forget your sit-ups for the next few months and do the following moderate but effective abdominal exercises.

The halfway curl-up

For strengthening the straight abdominal muscles.

Starting position:
Lie on back, arms alongside, legs comfortably apart with knees bent at 45-degree angle and feet firmly planted on floor.

Movements:
1. While slowly exhaling, press small of back to floor, raise arms slightly to reach forward and curl head and shoulders off the floor. Give little forward thrusts with your arms, starting about three times, to help you reach farther and to sustain the tension in your straight abdominal muscles. See Figure 3-12. Hold a moment.

Fig. 3-12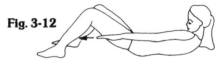

2. Then slowly uncurl, easing shoulders, head, and then arms to floor and inhale with relish.
3. Relax, allowing yourself time to breathe out and in deeply before starting again on an exhale. Don't rush. Breathing in between exercises is important.
4. Repeat 3-5 times.

The side-twist curl-up

For the crisscross abdominal muscles.

Starting position:
Same as for the halfway curl-up except that right arm is crossed over to the left, with left hand resting, palm down, on the outside of your left thigh.

Movements:

1. While s-l-o-w-l-y exhaling (sssssss), press small of back to floor, reach right hand forward along the outside of your left thigh, aiming for the front of your left knee, and curl head and right shoulder up off the floor, twisting them to the left. (Figure 3-13). Give three little thrusts with your right arm. Hold at the top for a count of three.

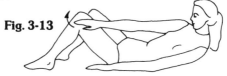

Fig. 3-13

2. Now slowly uncurl, returning right shoulder, right arm, and head to starting position, and inhale as head meets floor.
3. Relax and breathe out and in deeply before starting again on an exhale with your other arm.
4. Alternating arms, repeat 2-3 times with each arm.
5. Then, on an exhale, curl head and shoulders off the floor, and alternating arms, reach across from one side to the other in rapid succession for a slow count of 6, before slowly lowering yourself (with control) to starting position and inhaling deeply.
6. Do the side-twisting curl-up 2-3 times, always taking time out to relax and breathe naturally after each repeat.

The one-legged twist

For the crisscross abdominal muscles, the abductors of the inner thighs, hips, and spine flexibility.

Breathing instructions:
Inhale on movement 1 and exhale on movement 2.

Starting position:
Lie on back, arms extended sideways at shoulder level, palms down, left leg stretched out along the floor and right leg drawn up, bent at the knee with foot flat on the floor.

Movements:
1. Without lifting shoulders off the floor, cross your bent right knee over your straight leg, twisting pelvis to the left and touch right knee to floor, while turning your head in the opposite (right) direction (Figure 3-14a). (Feel the pull on your right side?)
2. Then swing bent knee back up and over straight leg and relax it outward to the floor on the right; rolling head around to the left (Figure 3-14b). (Feel the stretch in your groin on the right?)
3. Repeat steps 1 and 2 5-6 times with each leg, always turning your head in the opposite direction of your bent knee.
4. Now, for a slightly different pull on your abdominal muscles and an extra bottom firming effect, sit up, prop yourself up on your hands, with fingers pointed inward (Figure 3-14c) and do 3-5 more back and forth twists with each leg (Figure 3-14d).

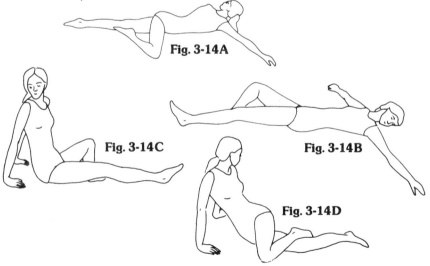

Fig. 3-14A

Fig. 3-14C

Fig. 3-14B

Fig. 3-14D

The side-lying shrug

For waist and hips and for limbering up the sacroiliac joints.

Breathing instructions:
Shrug on an exhale; stretch on an inhale.

Starting position:
Lie on your right side, propped up on your right elbow, with legs straight, one on top of the other and left arm curved gently over your upper thigh. Balance your lower body on your right hip.

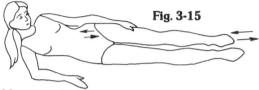

Fig. 3-15

Movements:

1. Tense and slightly raise your left leg, pointing toes (Figure 3-15).
2. Without leaning forward, rhythmically shrug and then stretch your left leg 6-8 times.
3. Roll over on your back to your left side and repeat the rhythmic shrug-s-t-r-e-t-c-h movement 6-8 more times with your right leg.
4. Rest a moment and then repeat once.

Important! *Remember to "hold" your belly as you roll from side to side.*

Waistline tucks

Breathing instructions:
Exhale as you reach down with your hand and inhale as you glide from side to side.

Starting position:
Lie on back, small of back naturally curved, hands straight along sides, and legs comfortably apart, with knees bent at a 45-degree angle and feet straight, flat on the floor.

Movements:

1. Without lifting head and body off the floor, reach right arm along floor to right foot, pulling head and torso sideways and tucking waistline in on the right (Figure 3-16a). Starting 3 or 4 times, give little rhythmic thrusts with your right

Fig. 3-16A

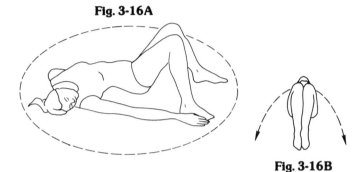

Fig. 3-16B

hand to help you reach farther, while exhaling on *sssssss*.

2. Return to starting position, smoothly gliding head and torso back up along the floor.
3. Then repeat on the left, keeping the movements fluid.
4. Moving from side to side in a smooth, uninterrupted arc, do 4-6 tucks on each side.
5. Finish off by returning to starting position and resting a moment, breathing naturally.
6. Then limber up by rolling your bent knees lazily around from side to side in a smooth uninterrupted arc (Figure 3-16b). Keep the pace fluid and easygoing, taking care to keep your legs together and your shoulders down on the floor.

The elevated body-roll

A multi-purpose abdominal exercise that strengthens all three groups of abdominal muscles.

Starting position:
Lie on your back, with legs together, bent at the knees at a 45-degree angle. Clasp your hands beneath your neck.

Movements:
1. Keeping head and shoulders down on the floor, inhale and gently drop both knees to the right, touching lower knee to floor while turning your head in the opposite direction of your knees, in this case to the left (Figure 3-17a).
2. Bounce knees lightly 3 times as you exhale. Then relax and inhale when you feel the need.
3. On your next exhale, curl head, shoulders, and arms up off the floor to look at the soles of your feet (Figure 3-17b). Hold for a count of 3.
4. Then slowly uncurl, easing first back, then shoulders, head and finally elbows to floor, and inhale deeply.
5. Repeat steps 3 and 4 two or three times.
6. Then exhale, press small of back to floor and swing bent knees up to starting position.
7. Repeat on your other side.

Tip: *Keep knees and feet together throughout the entire exercise.*

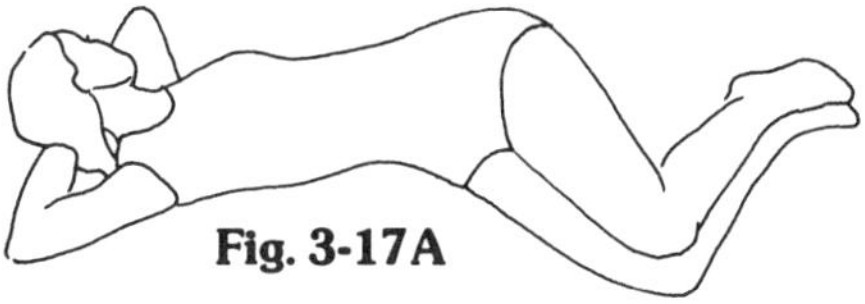

Fig. 3-17A 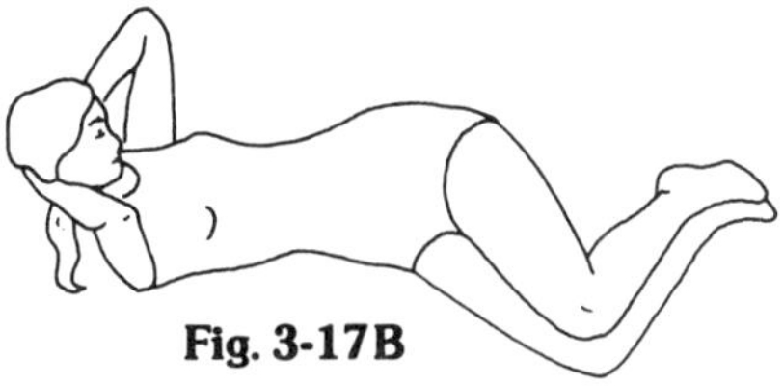   Fig. 3-17B

Don't be discouraged if you have difficulty curling head and shoulders forward at first. With practice it will come.

Now curl up slightly on your left side with your head resting on your left hand, your legs together, one on top of the other, knees bent and drawn up to waist level, and right hand resting on right knee. Breathe quietly for a moment, according to your own natural breathing rhythm. Then do the following dual-purpose breathing exercise:

The backstroke swing

A relaxing, chest-expanding breathing exercise that gently exercises the crisscross abdominal muscles.

Starting position:
As described above, illustrated in Figure 3-18a.

Movements:
1. On an inhale, swing right arm gracefully up and across to the right, moving it diagonally in a wide arc and turning your head to look at your swinging hand as you set it gently down, palm up, on the floor behind you, reaching only as far back as you can comfortably go. See Figure 3-18b.
2. Hold; exhale slowly and then inhale when you feel the need, filling your lungs to capacity.
3. On the next exhale, pull tummy firmly in toward spine and gracefully swing right arm and head back to starting position.

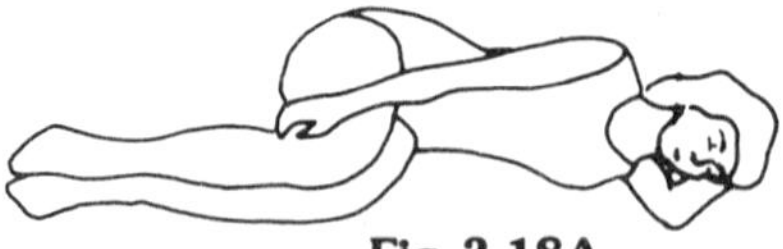

Fig. 3-18A 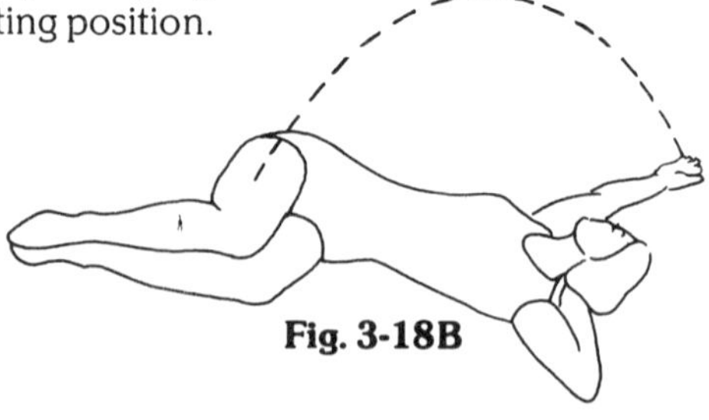   **Fig. 3-18B**

4. Repeat once or twice on the same side.
5. Then wrap one arm around your belly for support, roll over on your other side and do 2-3 more backstroke swings with your left arm.
6. End by remaining on your side and breathing quietly for a while with your eyes closed.

When you're ready, rise slowly in stages to a sitting position and complete your workout for the day by doing the sitting squat.

The sitting squat

Starting position:
Sit on the floor, knees bent wide apart with soles of feet touching and torso tilted slightly forward.

Movements:
1. Place hands on knees and press them gently down to floor (Figure 3-19a). Release and let knees bounce back.
2. Repeat 3-5 times.
3. Cross your hands and grasp your feet so that palm of right hand touches left foot and palm of left hand touches right foot (Figure 3-19b).
4. Keeping arms straight and torso tilted forward, aligned with head, bounce knees lightly several times.
5. On an exhale bend elbows out at the sides and, keeping back straight, lean forward as far as you can go *without* rounding your back (Figure 3-19c). Bounce 3 times to help you reach lower. Hold a moment and inhale before straightening arms and lifting head and torso into starting position.
6. Repeat step 5 2-3 times.

Note: *If you suffer from varicose veins squat sitting down rather than standing.*

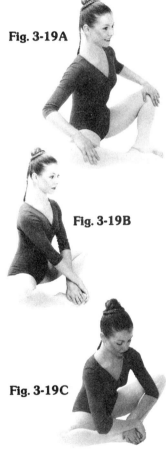

Fig. 3-19A

Fig. 3-19B

Fig. 3-19C

Chapter Four

EVERYTHING YOU NEED TO KNOW ABOUT VARICOSE VEINS

Although varicose veins acquired during pregnancy do tend to improve and even disappear after the birth, don't count on it! The walls of a vein are only slightly elastic to begin with, and once stretched they may not return to their pre-pregnancy condition. For this reason it is best to try and prevent varicose veins from developing in the first place.

Before going into the do's and don'ts of an all-round preventive plan, it helps to have a general understanding of the structure of a vein and the most common causes of a varicosity.

Simply stated, a vein is a tubular branching vessel that carries venous blood (blood depleted of oxygen and loaded with carbon dioxide and other wastes) back to the heart. Within the simple tube of the vein are many little valves, and surrounding the valves is a layer of interwoven elastic tissue fibers and smooth muscle cells. As they simultaneously contract and relax, the "milking" action of these muscles opens and shuts the valves, thereby pumping the blood toward the heart while hindering a backward clog-up of blood in the vein. (See Figure 4-1.)

In the feet, legs, and pelvis these muscles and valves work against the law of gravity, pumping the blood upward toward the heart. And that is where the problem lies.

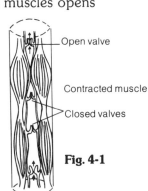

Open valve

Contracted muscle

Closed valves

Fig. 4-1

Merely standing for long periods of time can cause enough back pressure to enlarge the already thin vein walls. Once the walls are enlarged, the valves may become incompetent and the effect of gravity is then able to impede the upward flow of blood, causing a clog-up of blood in the veins, or, in other words, a varicosity.

During pregnancy, when your blood supply is increased and pregnancy hormones promote a general loosening up effect in your body, the walls of your veins are more likely to dilate and weaken than at any other time, especially if there is a history of varicose veins in your family. To make matters worse, all the veins which carry venous blood from the feet, legs, and pelvis back to the heart join up to form one large vessel in the pelvis, just behind the uterus: the inferior vena cava (Figure 4-9, page 86). When the expectant mother stands, the weight of her enlarged uterus and its contents may press against a certain area of this major vein, causing a "traffic block" of venous blood in her pelvic veins that impedes her circulation and causes back pressure right down her legs to her feet.

Fortunately, there *is* much that can be done (and a number of things that should *not* be done) to ward off, or at least limit, the development of unsightly, painful varicose veins and the many side effects which often result.

THE DO'S AND THE DON'TS

DON'T

1. Don't stand for long, uninterrupted periods of time.
2. Don't cross your legs at the knee. (This restricts the circulation in your legs.)
3. Don't sit back on your heels, or squat, except briefly while exercising.
4. Don't wear garters, half-length elastic stockings, knee-socks, or tight-fitting panties. (The elastic borders cut into the skin and impede the circulation in the legs.)

5. Don't take a hot bath or a sauna. (Heat promotes the expansion of the vein walls, which is the last thing you want to do!

6. Don't wear tight-fitting socks, very high heels, or shoes that pinch.

DO:

1. Do stimulate your circulation while standing and sitting by occasionally wiggling your toes, bending and stretching your ankles, and rolling your feet around in circles, clockwise and counterclockwise. (Many feet and leg exercises can be done while standing in the kitchen, sitting at a desk, etc.)

2. Do wear support stockings or pantyhose. For legs that ache, feel heavy, swell up, or are clouded with a faint network of blue lines under the skin, wear full-length two-way elastic stockings. Put them on in the morning on your *raised legs* before getting out of bed.

3. Do take time out to rest during the day, lying on your back with bottom propped up on a small pillow and legs raised diagonally, supported by a turned over chair (as shown in Figure 4-2); or rest your heels on a couch, bed, or any other stable furniture of similar height with legs stretched out loosely (as shown in Figure 4-3).

4. Do shift the weight of your baby off the vena cava and stimulate the upward flow of venous blood to the heart from leg and pelvic veins by getting down on your knees and elbows every now and then, with palms, forearms and

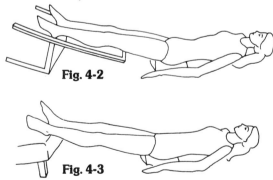

Fig. 4-2

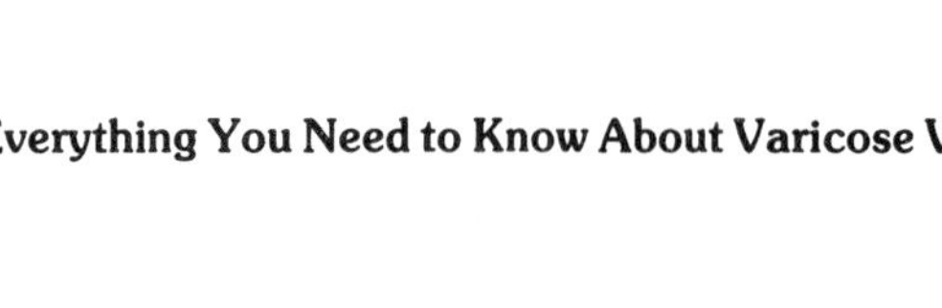

Fig. 4-3

elbows flat on the floor beneath your shoulders and knees directly under hips. This elbow-knee position is illustrated in Figure 4-4. Keep back straight, aligned with neck and head; don't sag at the waist.

For longer periods in this resting position, raise your forearms off the floor and "hold" your face in the palms of your hands, as shown in Figure 4-5. (Try reading in this position.)

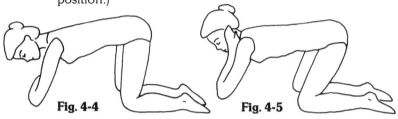

Fig. 4-4   Fig. 4-5

Tip: *During first-stage labor, either version of the kneeling elbow-knee resting position helps ease pressure felt in the lower back (back labor).*

5. Do go for brisk walks, making sure to maintain a good walking posture.
6. Do give yourself a quick, cold-water leg massage once or even twice a day, usually after removing your elastic stockings for your afternoon rest or before retiring at night. Use a hand shower attachment and massage one leg at a time (Figure 4-6), starting at the back of the toes and continuing upward along sole and calf to the back of the thigh, moving

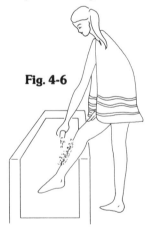

Fig. 4-6

in a quick circular pattern. Then start again in front, working upward from toes to instep, ankle, calf, knee, and thigh. This water massage stimulates the circulation, reduces swelling, eases pain, and helps tauten and improve the elasticity of the vein walls and the skin of the legs. It also leaves your legs tingling all over and delightfully warm. To keep the rest of you warm while you work on your legs, drape a towel over your shoulders and stand with one leg outside of the tub and one inside.

Note: *In hot weather, of if you already suffer from varicose veins, step up your cold water leg massage to 3 times daily.*

7. Do soothe heavy, aching, or swollen legs with a light fingertip massage at the end of a long day, always taking care not to massage directly on any existing varicosities. With gentle strokes, massage the raised leg, starting at the sole of the foot and working around the heel and upward along ankle, calf, and thigh.

8. Do bandage your legs for the night several times a week, or every night if you already have varicose veins. Using either long linen or cotton bandages* which have been soaked in cold water and then wrung out, *lightly* bind your feet and legs, starting at the instep and working up to either the knee or the thigh (depending on the condition of your legs). Then bind long, dry woolen bandages over the wet ones and fasten with little elastic clips; or else wear long 100 percent pure woolen stockings. Do this after you've gone to bed for the night and don't get up until you remove them in the morning! To keep the bandages from wetting your bed, keep a bath towel or bed protector under your legs while binding them and remove it immediately once dry bandages are in place.

9. Do tauten the skin of your legs—Nature's very own elastic stockings—by giving yourself a loofah or dry brush massage every now and then, moving upward along each leg in a slow circular pattern.

WARNING: No leg massages should be done when there is an inflammation of the veins.

*You can make them yourself from an old linen or cotton sheet.

10. Do raise the foot of your bed by 4 to 6 inches so that both legs and pelvis are elevated, furthering the upward flow of venous blood to the heart. Raising only the legs (as in Figure 4-7) is not sufficient, as the blood tends to get pooled in the pelvic veins. The proper incline is shown in Figure 4-8.
11. Do swim regularly in clean, cool water.
12. Do consult a physician if you have pain, swelling, ulcers, or blotches on your legs!
13. Do exercise daily (following the exercise plan given in this chapter) to stimulate the circulation in the veins of the pelvis and legs and indirectly massage some of the superficial veins. Start with the toes and work your way upward in accordance with the anatomical sequence of vein groups involved: leg veins, pelvic veins and the inferior vena cava (see Figure 4-9).

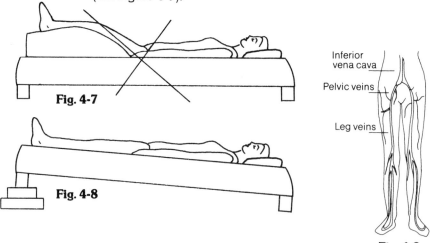

Fig. 4-7

Fig. 4-8

Inferior vena cava

Pelvic veins

Leg veins

Fig. 4-9

If all of this sounds like a great deal of bother, just ask any woman who has varicose veins what she wouldn't do to be rid of them.

The following anti-varicosity exercise program is taught in Switzerland at many maternity gymnastic classes and has successfully helped to prevent, lessen, and limit varicose veins for many expectant mothers (myself included).

THE ANTI-VARICOSITY PROGRAM

WAKING-UP EXERCISES
Do the three simple exercises in this section first thing in the morning, before getting out of bed. If you already suffer from varicose veins, or if the condition tends to run in your family, do them at least twice a day: once in the morning (before putting on your elastic stockings) and once again at night, after retiring. Don't despair. All together they take less than 4 minutes to do.

The 90-second leg workout
For stimulating circulation in the entire leg, strengthening leg and foot muscles (especially at the arch), and indirectly massaging some of the superficial veins.

Note: *No matter how difficult it may be to carry out this entire exercise—don't give up! Keep going until a full 90 seconds are up. It gets easier with practice. Time yourself. Steps 2 to 5 should take exactly 30 seconds and step 6 exactly 15 seconds. All movements should be kept rhythmic, with the tempo gradually quickening and then slowing down again.*

Starting position:
Lie on your back, at the edge of your bed, with both legs bent at a 45-degree angle.

Movements:
1. Stretch the leg nearest to the edge up straight, with toes pointed to ceiling (Figure 4-10a).

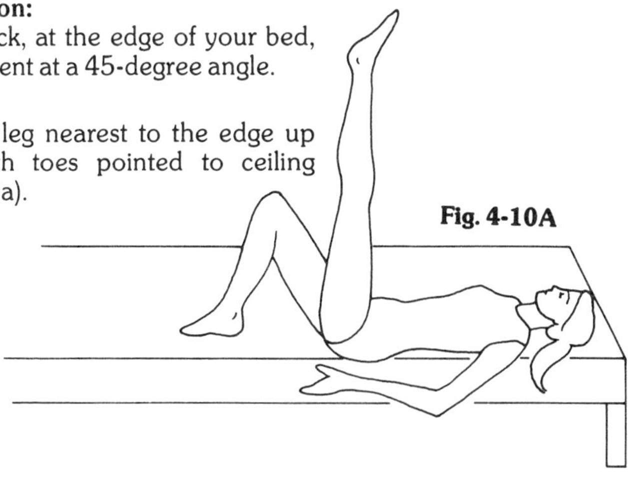

Fig. 4-10A

2. Keeping raised knee very straight, firmly bend and stretch toes of extended leg (Figure 4-10b). Start slowly and keep the movements rhythmic, gradually increasing in speed and vigor, and then slowing down again.

Fig. 4-10B

3. Bend and stretch ankle so that first heel and then toes point to ceiling (Figure 4-10c). *Feel* the stretch and gradually work up to a faster tempo, then slow down.

Fig. 4-10C

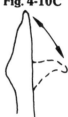

4. Bend ankle and turn foot from side to side (in-out-in-out) keeping up the familiar slow-fast-slow tempo (Figure 4-10d). (Don't forget to keep knee straight!)
5. Roll foot around in circles (clockwise and counterclockwise) keeping the arc as wide as possible (Figure 4-10e) and maintaining the changing pace of tempo until the first 30 seconds are up. Then, in a smooth continuous motion . . .

Fig. 4-10D

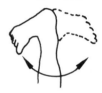

6. . . . drop leg over edge of bed (keeping knee straight) and continue to rotate foot as in step 5, alternating direction and speed for another 15 seconds (Figure 4-10f).
7. Then, quickly swing leg up straight as at start, keeping toes pointed and knee straight, and repeat steps 2 to 6 for another 45 seconds.

Fig. 4-10E

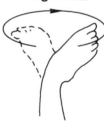

8. Move over to opposite edge of bed and repeat the leg workout with your other leg for another full 90 seconds.

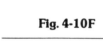

Fig. 4-10F

The gentle leg-shakedown

A limbering-up exercise, which also helps relieve circulatory congestion in the legs.

Starting position:
Lie on back, hands along sides and knees bent at a 45-degree angle.

Movements:

1. Slowly extend right leg up until it is almost, but not quite, vertical, with knee slightly flexed and toes pointed.
2. Gently vibrate raised leg (Figure 4-11), while turning heel slightly in and out. *Feel* the vibration up in your toes and right down to your thigh.
3. Slowly lower leg to starting position and repeat with other leg.

Note: *Don't shake leg vigorously.*

Fig. 4-11

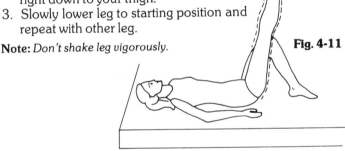

The partial kickup

For strengthening leg muscles (especially those which act upon the knee joint) and stimulating the circulation in the legs.

Starting position:
Lie on back, arms along sides, knees bent, and feet planted firmly on the bed.

Movements:

1. Stretch one leg upward until it is straight and at right angles to bed, with knee straight and toes pointed to ceiling (Figure 4-12a).

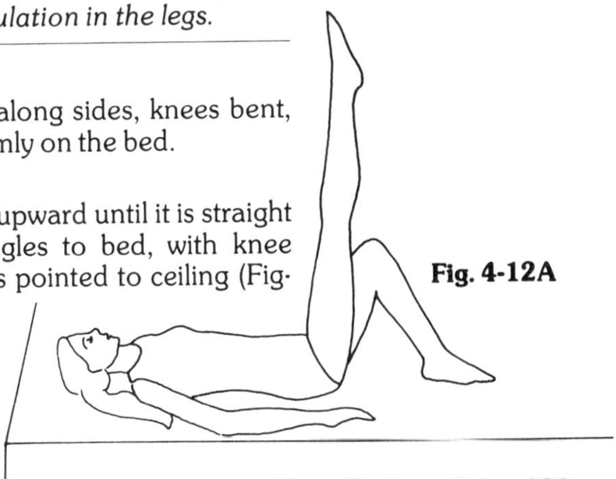

Fig. 4-12A

2. Tense leg from toes to top of thigh. Hold for a moment.
3. Then abruptly drop calf, letting it hang down limply from the joint while keeping thigh up (Figure 4-12b).
4. Kick calf up, straightening knee, pointing toes, and stretching leg as tall as it will go.
5. Hold for a moment, then repeat exercise 3-5 times.
6. Do the same with your other leg.

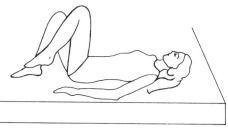

Fig. 4-12B

ADDITIONAL ANTI-VARICOSITY EXERCISES

If you consider yourself a likely candidate for varicose veins, or if you already suffer from the condition or from swollen, painful legs, do the two exercises in this section at least once a day. Choose whatever time suits you best.

Upside-down scissors

For stimulating circulation in the legs and in the external iliac veins running through the groin. It also helps keep the abductor muscles pliant and supple.

Starting position:
Lie down in front of a wall with buttocks pressed against it and stretch your legs straight up along the wall.

Movements:
1. Warm up by rhythmically bending and stretching toes, moving feet back and forth, in and out, and around in circles, both clockwise and counter-clockwise, *without* lifting heels off wall.
2. Point toes and glide one leg sideways along wall, bringing it down to rest on the floor, or as far as it will go (Figure 4-13a).

3. Relax; wait until your lowered leg feels warm (from the onrush of fresh blood coursing through the veins). Then tighten leg and seat muscles and slowly glide lowered leg back up to center.
4. Do the same with other leg.
5. Alternating legs, repeat steps 2 to 4, 2-3 times, ending with legs in starting position.
6. Finish by scissoring legs as wide as comfortable (Figure 4-13b)—pausing—and then slowly returning both legs to center, simultaneously. Repeat this step 1-2 times.
7. Curl up comfortably on your side, with knees drawn up and elbows bent, and rest for a moment before moving on to the next exercise.

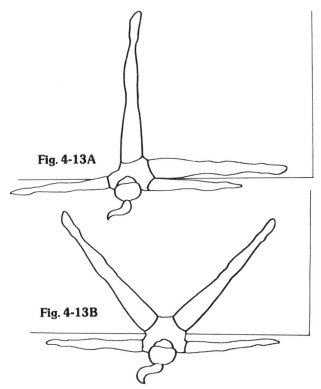

Fig. 4-13A

Fig. 4-13B

Spine rolling

For relieving pressure on pelvic veins, assisting the return of venous blood to the heart from legs and pelvis, strengthening abdominal and pelvic floor muscles, and keeping spine flexibile.

Starting position:
Lie on back, arms straight along sides, palms down, knees comfortably parted and bent at a 45-degree angle, with feet straight and flat on the floor or bed.

Movements:
1. While exhaling, simultaneously draw in lower abdomen (directly above pubic bones), tighten pelvic floor muscles and tuck seat under, pressing small of back firmly to floor and tilting pelvis up, so that buttocks rise slightly off the floor. Chin sinks to chest.
2. Using feet for leverage, slowly ease back up off the floor, one vertebra at a time, until body rests entirely on shoulders and feet (Figure 4-14).

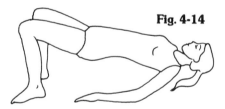

Fig. 4-14

3. Pause at the top to breathe in slowly and deeply.
4. When you feel the need, let your breath out as you pull tummy firmly in and tighten seat and pelvic floor.
5. Still maintaining your raised position, inhale slowly and deeply.
6. Then exhale; pull tummy in, tighten seat and pelvic floor, and very cautiously ease

back down to floor in a slow, catlike motion, feeling each vertebra as it meets the floor.
7. Inhale and relax, letting spine return to its natural arch at waist level (small of back).
8. Follow up with some gentle spine-swinging. (See page 37).
9. Repeat 2-3 more times.
10. Now roll over and rest on your side with elbows and knees flexed. Close your eyes and relax, breathing naturally for a moment or two. Then rise slowly in stages and open your eyes.

Fig. 4-15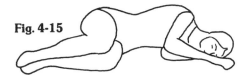

Tip: *Whether your legs are flawless after the birth of your baby or whether they are marked with a network of blue veins, continue to exercise your legs for at least the first six postpartum weeks, or for as long as you breastfeed. If you wore two-way stretch elastic stockings during pregnancy, continue wearing them for the first few postpartum weeks; eventually switch to light support stockings or pantyhose to help you adjust to going without the support of elastic stockings.*

Chapter Five

PREPARING FOR NURSING

The very first time you put your baby to your breast you may be shocked at the force of his or her suck. As every nursing mother knows, each baby comes with his own built-in technique and tempo, but most take to their task at once with instant enthusiasm and expertise.

Whatever your baby's approach, one thing is certain: he'll be far too intent on satisfying his own needs to show any regard for your tender nipples. Caring for them is entirely up to you—and the sooner you start the better. With a little know-how and perseverance you can prevent sore, cracked, and even flat nipples from marring an otherwise perfect beginning to a lifelong relationship.

So, if you're planning to nurse, or even if you're just toying with the idea, make it a point to add the following conditioning measures to your daily routine. They take only a few minutes of each day—a small investment for such high dividends.

To harden your nipples and make them easier for your baby to grasp, practice the following procedures, starting as early as possible in your pregnancy.

Note: *To protect the delicate tissues of your breasts, always cup the breast being exercised or massaged with the palm of the hand on the same side and work with the other hand.*

The rub-down

Lightly pass a rough, dry washcloth over your nipple several times, moving up and down and around in circles. Repeat with other nipple. After two to three months of this daily massage, replace the washcloth with a soft toothbrush and gently "brush" each nipple from side to side and around in circles.

The pull-up
Especially beneficial for flat nipples.

Place fingertips of thumb, index, and middle finger around the nipple. Keeping these three fingers stiff, press fingertips into the areola (the dark area around the nipple). Grasp the nipple firmly and pull it out as far as it can go. Then, still grasping the nipple, press fingers back down into the areola. Repeat about 5 in-and-out movements, always making sure to keep the three working fingers stiff. Do the same with your other breast.

The nipple twist

Using the same three fingers as in the pull-up, grasp the nipple, pull it out and twist it firmly two times to the right, in a corkscrew motion, and then two times to the left. Repeat 3-5 times in each direction with each nipple.

Keeping nipples dry

Expose your nipples to the air every now and then and, if possible, to sunlight, starting with a very brief exposure.

Correcting inverted nipples

For truly inverted nipples wear Woolwich breast shields. Originally from England, these shields can now be obtained in the United States. To find out where, contact the La Leche League branch nearest to you. In fact, even if you aren't troubled by inverted nipples it's advisable to get in touch with this organization of experienced nursing mothers for additional information—with a personal touch.

Oiling

Except for the last few weeks of your pregnancy, follow up your nipple routine either by oiling the nipples with almond oil, olive oil, etc., or by applying vaseline or pure lanolin.

In addition to keeping your nipples fit for nursing take care to keep yourself in form for the strain nursing places on shoulders, back, and breasts. Spend two minutes of every day doing the simple, but effective, chest-arm-shoulder exercises listed in Program B. You can do them in the morning, while sitting on the edge of your bed.

II

THE COPING TECHNIQUES

A do-it-yourselves guide for expectant parents learning the Swiss method

Chapter Six

UNDERSTANDING LABOR "PAINS"

A contraction is often compared to a wave which grows stronger and stronger as it swells to a crest and then weakens as it falls back into the sea, while a woman in labor is comparable to a lone swimmer in a stormy sea. If she panics and runs, she is bound to be overtaken and pulled under by the waves. But if she swims confidently toward them and "rides" the waves, she can keep her head above the water. Being able to do this takes timing, know-how, and self-control.

Just like the swimmer, you need adequate preparation in order to be able to "ride the waves" of labor confidently. If you learn to understand what actually happens within your body during a contraction, and if you master certain breathing and relaxation techniques, you will be able to accept your contractions and "breathe over" them, knowing that each one is bringing you closer to your goal: the natural birth of your baby.

The mother who is unprepared, however, is frightened by the unfamiliar sensations of uterine muscular contraction and instinctively protects herself from each oncoming wave by tensing up and cramping her muscles, unwittingly adding to the intensity of her contractions. Her fear also affects the rate of her breathing—making it rapid and shallow as when in flight.

Don't let this happen to you! The age-old fear of labor pains is greatly reduced if you can appreciate the intricate, well-coordinated efforts being made by your uterine muscles to pull open the "door" of your womb and send your baby safely out on its way.

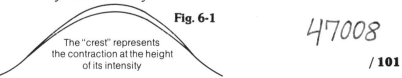

Fig. 6-1

The "crest" represents the contraction at the height of its intensity

47008

THE PHYSIOLOGY OF FIRST-STAGE LABOR (THE DILATION STAGE)

Labor means hard work, but during the first stage of labor it's the uterus—not the mother—that should be doing all of the hard physical work. When the uterine muscles contract during this stage of labor, the upper segment (the major, thicker portion of the uterus) contracts most strongly, growing shorter and thicker, while the thinner, circular muscle fibers of the lower segment (the lowest part of the uterine body and the cervix, which is the mouth of the uterus) contract only mildly and stretch, becoming thinner and thinner. As the cervix thins out, it is eventually "taken up" into the body of the uterus and pulled open. In the intervals between contractions the muscles relax but the upper segment does not regain its former length. Instead it remains a little bit shorter and thicker and is able to apply somewhat more pressure on the baby with the next contraction. In this way the uterine muscles work together during every contraction to force the baby lower down into the pelvis and at the same time to thin and open the cervix and pull it up over the baby's head (or breach).

THE MOTHER'S ROLE DURING FIRST STAGE LABOR

During this stage of labor the mother who is able consciously to relax and remain physically passive, yet mentally aware and in control of her breathing, supports her uterus in its efforts and supplies it with the oxygen it needs to work efficiently.

On the other hand, the mother who is tense and physically active unwittingly opposes the dilation of her cervix and causes herself unnecessary pain.

To understand why this is so, we need to consider the following:
1. Oxygen, taken from the bloodstream, is the fuel that muscles need to work.
2. Whenever a muscle contracts, fuel (oxygen) is burned, leaving a residue of waste and carbon dioxide.

3. When the muscle relaxes, these "wastes" are washed away by the bloodstream and replaced with freshly oxygenated blood.
4. For as long as the muscle remains tensed to even the slightest degree, blood vessels are being squeezed, slowing down the circulation to and from that muscle, and leaving the waste to accumulate.
5. If the waste products of muscular activity are not removed fast enough due to poor circulation, they can cause severe pain.*

Fig. 6-2

Uterus at start of labor

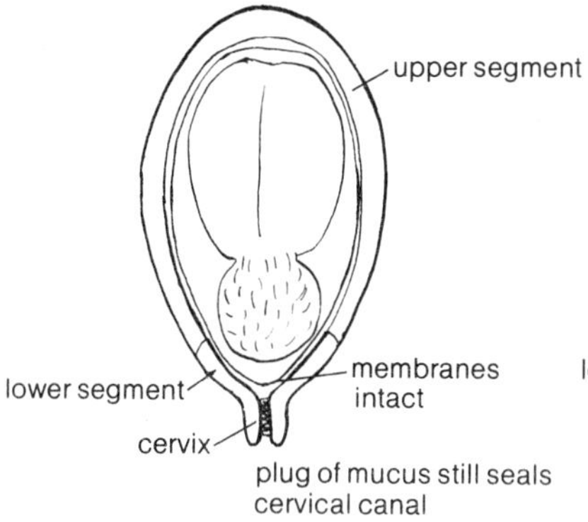

upper segment

lower segment

cervix

membranes intact

plug of mucus still seals cervical canal

Fig. 6-3

Cervix taken up but not dilated

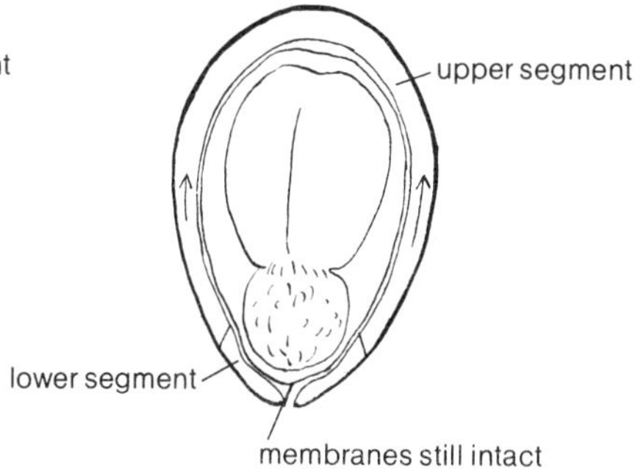

upper segment

lower segment

membranes still intact

Fig. 6-4

Cervix is dilating

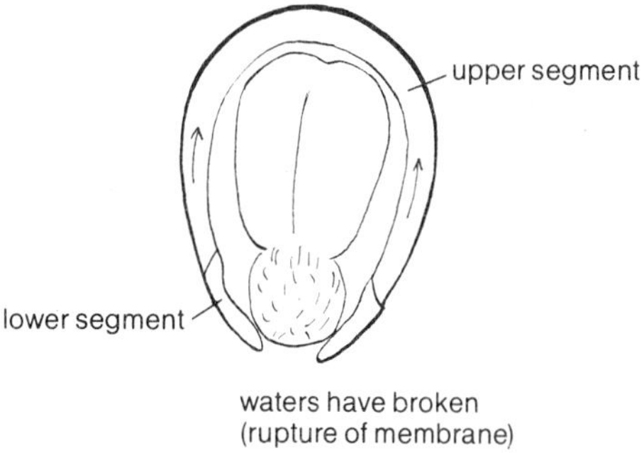

upper segment

lower segment

waters have broken (rupture of membrane)

*A classic example of this is angina pectoris; the lack of oxygen to the heart muscle causes severe pain.

Therefore, if the mother relaxes all those muscles which can be consciously controlled, and releases all mental tension (which automatically translates into muscular tension), circulation is centered in the pelvic area, where the action is. Furthermore, maintaining a state of relaxation in between as well as during contractions enables the uterus to relax fully after contracting. Now the blood can rush in through the dilated blood vessels and carry away the wastes while supplying the hard-working uterine muscles with the oxygen-rich blood they need.

Summed up: Relaxation during the first stage of labor, on both a physical and emotional plane, reduces pain, promotes the unhampered progression of labor, and conserves the mother's energy for later on, when she will need it to push her baby out into the world.

In light of all this, it is not surprising that most women using the deep, trancelike relaxation and the quiet, soothing "graduated" breathing taught in Switzerland have been known to have significantly easier and shorter labors.

To improve your chances of coping calmly and effectively during childbirth, from start to finish, study the Swiss-styled coping techniques found in this section (Part II). For best results, give yourself ample time to learn and thoroughly master all of the given coping techniques at a leisurely pace, instead of planning a quick (and risky) "crash course" at the end of your pregnancy. To help you chart your own training program study the recommended schedule opposite.

GENERAL OUTLINE FOR LEARNING THE COPING TECHNIQUES

SUBJECT	IDEAL TIME TO START	BEGINNERS	ADVANCED
Relaxation	In the first trimester	a. Practice the preliminary exercises often, at any convenient, peaceful time of day or night. **Tip:** Relaxation is easier to learn following an invigorating workout.	a. Practice deep-conscious relaxation once every day, preferably at night in bed, just before falling asleep. b. From time to time practice while the father (or any other helper) reads the instructions aloud.
Breathing	In the second trimester	a. Unless otherwise specified in the instructions, limit yourself to one new breathing exercise (not counting preliminary exercises) per week and keep at it, practicing often, for short periods until you have mastered it. b. As you advance from one breathing technique to the next review the "old" ones by practicing them briefly once or twice a week.	Polish up your newly acquired breathing skills by: a. Making it a habit to practice a different breathing technique for a minute or two during the day whenever you get the chance (i.e. while riding the subway, filing your nails, washing dishes, etc.) b. 2-3 times a week "rehearse" breathing over labor contractions, using the various breathing techniques in turn. The father can help by timing the contractions.
Pushing	In the third trimester	a. After mastering the preliminary exercises, make it a habit to practice pushing during every bowel movement. b. Practice pushing in the various pushing positions, 2 or 3 times a week.	a. Continue to practice your push daily during elimination. b. 2-3 times a week rehearse pushing with stops and starts while the father calls out the shots in turn (as described on page 165).

Chapter Seven

RELAXATION: THE SWISS WAY

Relaxation is "letting go"—beginning with the release of mental tension and anxiety and culminating in the physical release of muscular tension.

Because the ability to relax during labor is half the battle, the heart of the Swiss method is the relaxation program.

For best results, practice regularly throughout your entire pregnancy and pay attention to the following:

1. The room in which you practice should be well ventilated, but warm enough to be comfortable.
2. Turn off the lights and draw the shades the first few times you practice, in order to induce complete concentration.
3. In cold weather, cover yourself with a light blanket, sweater, coat, or any other light covering.
4. Make yourself comfortable. Remember that during labor you should be settled down comfortably enough to remain in the same position for a considerable length of time.

SUGGESTED POSITIONS FOR RELAXING

THE BACK-LYING (SUPINE) POSITION

Lie on your back with a pillow under your head and your legs comfortably apart with knees raised by a rolled-up pillow (or neck-roll) so that feet fall naturally outward on heels. Bend elbows slightly and open your hands. See Figure 7-1. This

Fig. 7-1

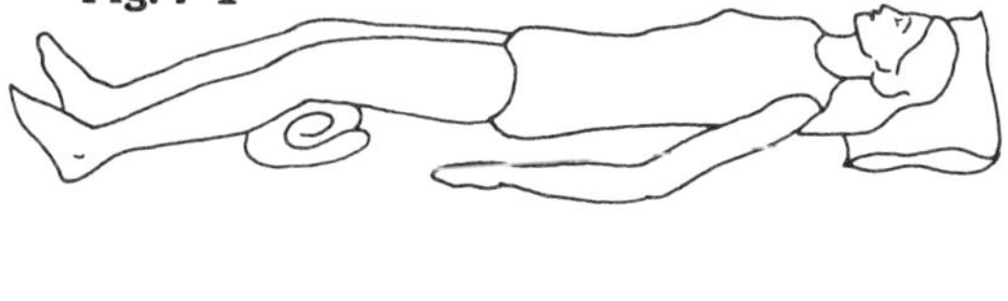

position is best suited for the early months of pregnancy since lying flat on your back during the later months and during the first stage of labor may result in supine-hypotension.*

THE SIDE-LYING (LATERAL) POSITION

Curl up slightly on whichever side seems more comfortable, making sure to lie on your *hip* (not your belly!) with your back well rounded and your head curled forward, resting on the lower edge of your pillow. Rest your lower arm behind you, bent loosely at the elbow, and draw the upper arm up in front so that hand rests at about eye level. Both legs should be bent at the knees, with the knee of the frontal leg up to your chest and supported by a folded pillow. See Figure 7-2.

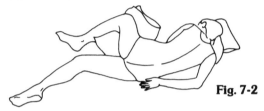

Fig. 7-2

Tip: *If you feel uncomfortable in this position due to pressure on the lower breast, cup the breast in the palm of your hand and draw it gently forward. Placing an extra pillow under your head also helps.*

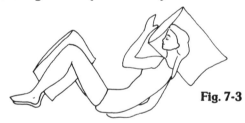

Fig. 7-3

Occasionally a woman finds lying on her side more comfortable with both knees drawn up and a pillow or two between her legs, as illustrated in Figure 7-3. If you use this position take care that the pillow under your head is high enough to

*Feeling faint and breathless when lying on the back due to pressure on the inferior vena cava by the pregnant uterus.

prevent your under shoulder from digging into the bed or other underlying surface, yet low enough to prevent an ache in your neck.

THE FORWARD-LEANING POSITION

During early labor this position is usually used at home and on the way to the hospital. You can do it sitting backwards on a chair with head and folded arms resting on the chair back (Figure 7-4) or sitting in the front seat of a car and leaning over the dashboard. To use this position while standing, spread feet comfortably apart, lean forward, and rest head and folded arms on some stable piece of furniture that is above waist height.

Whichever position you use always take special care to do the following:

1. Remove eyeglasses, bulky jewelry, etc.
2. Loosen tight clothing.
3. Close eyes and mouth lightly so that forehead is velvety smooth and jaws are loose.
4. Relax tongue and mouth.

Fig. 7-4

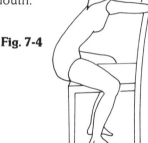

Before you even attempt to attain a state of deep conscious relaxation, you should learn to recognize the many fine sensations of tension which are always present, to some extent, whenever a muscle is tensed. To do this, practice the following "contrast" relaxation exercises, and experience for yourself the difference between a contracted and a relaxed muscle.

PRELIMINARY RELAXATION EXERCISES

Contrast Relaxation Exercise

Tip for beginners: *Have your husband (or a helper) read the instructions to you the first few times, or else record them on a tape recorder and play then back while you practice.*

Position:
Lie on your back with knees bent and supported by either a long or a folded pillow approximately 10 inches in diameter. Your eyes should be closed loosely and your body relaxed.

Movements:
1. Raise right arm slightly up off the mat, floor, bed, or whatever you are lying on.
2. Tightly clench right hand into a fist. Then stretch and tense the entire arm from wrist to shoulder.
3. Hold the tension for a few seconds and think: "My right arm is tensed."
4. Abruptly relax your arm and let it flop down. Feel how heavy it is as it sinks down, even deeper onto the mat.
5. Repeat with your left arm and then with both arms simultaneously.
6. Now lift your right calf slightly up off the mat without losing contact with the pillow under your knee.
7. Then stretch and tense the entire leg, from the hip to the tips of your toes.
8. Hold and feel the tension in your leg. (Think: "My right leg is tensed.")
9. Abruptly relax the leg, letting the calf flop down, pulled by its own weight.
10. Simultaneously tense your right arm and your left leg, in the manner already described.

11. Hold the tension a few seconds and check: Is your left arm still limp? Is your right leg limp?
12. Repeat with the alternate arm and leg; then with both arms and legs.
13. Keeping body still, hunch shoulders, bringing them up to your ears. Hold a moment. Then relax.
14. Press your head down into your pillow (floor, etc.). Press harder and harder. Then relax.

Another preliminary exercise which is essential for obtaining a true state of relaxation is conscious facial relaxation.

Facial Relaxation Exercise

1. Raise your eyebrows and wrinkle up your forehead.
2. Let them go slack—your forehead is smooth and wrinkle-free.
3. Frown, feel the tension.
4. Then let go gently and feel your forehead grow wide and smooth.
5. Open your eyes up wide, as if startled.
6. Let your eyes go slack and feel your eyelids grow heavy as they slowly close over your eyes.
7. Squint.
8. Then relax and feel your eyelids go loose.
9. Screw up your nose.
10. Then let it go loose.
11. Draw your nose downwards.
12. Relax it.
13. Clench jaws and bite down hard. Feel the tension.
14. Let go, and feel your cheeks sagging and your neck relax.
15. Tightly pucker up your lips.
16. Hold for a moment and then let your lips go slack.
17. Smile very broadly.
18. Hold your "smile" for a moment. Then let it go.
19. Stick your tongue out until it reaches almost to your chin.

20. Then slowly let your tongue slip back and rest in your mouth.
21. Press your chin down hard against your chest, straining your head forward.
22. Feel the tension mounting in your head, neck, and shoulders. Then stop pressing and relax.
23. Finish off by tensing all the muscles of your face at once and then relaxing them. Feel the tension draining from your face and neck. Don't rush. Give yourself time to experience the delightful relaxation of your smooth, expressionless face.

PELVIC FLOOR RELAXATION EXERCISES

Exercising your pelvic floor muscles regularly during pregnancy makes it easier for you to relax them during labor and delivery and improves the ability of these muscles to stretch easily during childbirth and recoil quickly afterwards.

Pelvic Floor Relaxation Exercise

Starting position:
Lie on your back with legs raised, bent at the knees, and hands clasped around the inner sides of your ankles so that feet are held up in midair (Figure 7-5).

Fig. 7-5

Movements:
1. Inhale and relax the pelvic floor muscles. (You should feel yourself "opening up" down below.)
2. Exhale slowly (*sssss*) and contract the muscles of the pelvic floor one by one as follows:
    a. tighten seat muscles;
    b. close the anus as if to check a bowel movement;
    c. tighten vagina and perineum (the area between anus and vagina);

    d. close the urethra, as it to stop
       the flow of urine in midstream;
    e. pull in your lower abdominal
       wall (directly above the pubic
       bones).
3. Hold the tension until all the air has been
   expelled from your lungs and you feel
   the *need* to inhale.
4. Inhale and slowly relax your pelvic floor
   muscles, one by one.
5. Repeat at least once, relaxing your pelvic
   floor muscles abruptly this time, instead
   of slowly.

DEEP-CONSCIOUS RELAXATION*

Now that you've learned to appreciate the difference between a tensed and a relaxed muscle and have acquired a certain skill for letting go and consciously releasing tension in isolated muscles, you are ready to learn deep-conscious relaxation.

    Begin by practicing together: you settled down comfortably on the floor (or any other hard, supporting surface), and your husband sitting nearby, dictating the instructions, which are given in the form of a text, in a low, soothing tone of voice. If you must practice alone in the beginning, record the following text on a tape recorder and play it back while you practice.

Deep-Conscious Relaxation Exercise

Position:
Settle down comfortably on your side (see side-lying position in Figure 7-2) in a darkened room. Close your eyes, relax your face, and try to clear your mind of all worries and thoughts. You'll need all your powers of concentration to relax every part of your

---

*Adapted from the principles of Autogenic Training, taught by Prof. J. H. Schultz of Berlin, and Eutonie Training, taught by Gerda Alexander of Copenhagen.

body and let yourself sink deep down and be carried by the underlying surface, like a log floating on water. (The following text assumes you are lying on your right side. If you aren't then simply change the instructions accordingly.)

Text:

"Relaxation is the art of letting go. Have no fear. Just let go-o-o and allow yourself to be carried by the underlying floor, rug, etc. You know your exact weight. Be conscious of every pound and ounce and let yourself sink deep, deep, down into the floor. Concentrate on your facial muscles. Your eyelids should be loose, your forehead wide and velvety smooth. Your jaws and cheeks should sag, your lips should be limp and, if you prefer, somewhat parted. Your tongue should be heavy" . . . PAUSE . . . "Just to be certain that your tongue and mouth are truly relaxed, press your tongue firmly against the roof of your mouth. Press harder, and even harder! *Feel* the tension mounting in your mouth, your neck, and down to your chest. Now let your tongue go slack and sink down, like a dead weight, toward the lower teeth on your right. Feel how heavy your tongue is, and how hollow and vast your mouth cavity is. Bear in mind that when your mouth and tongue are loose and relaxed, your vagina and cervix are also loose and relaxed." . . . PAUSE . . . "Now focus all your concentration on the inner side of your upper (left) foot. There where your foot touches the supporting surface—connect with it. Concentrate intensely on this spot, until you feel a current flowing out of your foot and down into the underlying surface." . . . PAUSE . . . "Once this is accomplished, focus all your concentration on the knee of your left leg. Exactly there where your knee touches your pillow, make contact." . . . PAUSE . . . "Be conscious of the entire weight of your left leg. *Feel* how heavy it is and let your knee sink deep down into the pillow." . . . PAUSE . . . "Now, concentrate on all those points where your left leg touches the underlying surface, and connect with it." . . . PAUSE . . . "Once you have succeeded, focus your entire concentration on the foot of your right leg. Exactly there where your foot comes in contact with the supporting surface, *connect* with it. Connect so intensely that you actually feel a current flowing out of your right foot and into the floor." . . . PAUSE . . . "Then, with all your innermost powers of concentration, continue along the calf, to the knee and thigh. Be conscious of all those points at which your right leg touches the floor and *bind* yourself to it." ... PAUSE ... "When you have successfully accomplished all this, focus your concentration on your right hip—the heaviest part of your body."... PAUSE ... "Check: Is your left hip also relaxed? Let g-o- under your hip bones—and feel the entire contents of your heavy pelvis sink down toward your right hip and into the underlying floor. Feel how heavy your right hip is, and let it sink deep, deep down into the floor."... PAUSE ... "Now, with your innermost powers of concentration, travel along the right contours of your torso, from your belly to your waist, and up to your breast cage. Wherever your torso touches the floor establish contact!" ... PAUSE ... "Check: Is the raised side of your breast cage slack? L-e-t g-o- under your collarbones. L-e-t g-o- in between your ribs. Be conscious of the weight of your breast cage, with all its contents. There where your breast cage touches the underlying surface, let the entire heavy contents of your chest sink deep, deep down into the floor." ... PAUSE ... "Once you have successfully accomplished all this, focus all your attention on your right shoulder. There where your right shoulder touches the underlying floor, connect with it." ... PAUSE ... "With your innermost powers of concentration, continue along your right arm, from the upper part of your arm to the lower part of your arm, and on to the back of your wrist and hand. Be conscious of all those areas where your right arm and hand touch the underlying surface, and make contact. Feel your heavy right arm sinking farther down into the floor. Concentrate on the back of your right hand. There where the back of your hand touches the floor, *connect* with it and feel the warmth flowing out of your hand and down into the floor. Now concentrate on the inside of your right hand, which is open and loose. *Feel* the warmth of your blood circulating in the very tips of your fingers." ... PAUSE ... "Now, focus all your concentration on your other arm, the one resting limply in front. Travel along this arm, from the shoulder to the elbow and on to the wrist. Wherever your left arm touches the floor (or the pillow), *connect* with it. L-e-t g-o under your left shoulder and feel the entire weight of your heavy left arm sinking down even deeper into the supporting surface." ... PAUSE ... "Now concentrate on your left hand, which is open and loose. Should your fingers touch the floor (or pillow), connect with it and feel the warm current flowing out of them and down into the supporting surface. If your fingers don't touch the underlying surface, concentrate on the blood circling in the tips of your fingers, warming them." ... PAUSE ... "When you have succeeded in accomplishing all this, focus your concentration on your neck and head. There where your head rests on your pillow, blend together with it. L-e-t g-o- under your ears. L-e-t g-o- under the base of your skull. Feel your head sinking even farther down into your pillow. *Unite* with your pillow and feel the current flowing out of your head and into your pillow." . . . PAUSE . . . "Make one last check of your face muscles. Are your jaws and cheeks sagged? Are your lips limp? Does your tongue drop like a dead weight against the teeth set in your right jaw." . . . . . . PAUSE . . . . . . (Father pauses quietly for a moment before adding the following positive suggestion) "And so you lie, completely relaxed and in contact with the supporting surface. Just as you will lie during labor, relaxed and at peace, calmly and confidently awaiting your next contraction, secure in the knowledge that with each one, you are helping the cervix open up for your baby and coming one step nearer to holding him or her in your arms. . . ."

Never rise straight up following a deep-conscious relaxation exercise. Either fall asleep right there where you are or else do the following snapping-back exercise to help stimulate your slowed-down blood circulation. Here, too, the father can help at first by calling out the movements in a loud, brisk tone of voice.

Snapping-back exercise

Note: *All movements should be gradually accelerated and then slowed down again.*

Movements:
1. Tightly clench hands into fists. Then open them wide, spreading fingers out with such intensity that palms and fingers turn white. Repeat several times, going faster and faster. Then slow down and stop.
2. Move hands up and down several times, and then around in circles, clockwise and counterclockwise.
3. Bending at the ankles, move feet forcefully back and forth several times, and then around in circles in both directions. Then shake them vigorously.

4. Breathe deeply, according to your natural breathing rhythm.
5. Then s-t-r-e-t-c-h, yawn, and prop yourself up on your elbow.
6. Sit up and open your eyes.
7. Rise slowly in stages.

Continue to practice deep-conscious relaxation with the father
from time to time, occasionally reversing roles. But, make it a
point to also practice regularly on your own, preferably at
night in bed, just before falling asleep.

Chapter Eight

CONTROLLED BREATHING: THE NATURAL ANESTHESIA

The way a woman breathes during labor makes a difference. It's not just a question of mind over matter. Certain breathing techniques actually alleviate pain on a physiological basis, and others don't. The problem is knowing which type of breathing to use and when to use it.

Some childbirth educators are staunch advocates of rhythmic chest breathing, which is distracting and inhibits the perception of pain; others are firm believers in the advantages of abdominal breathing and the benefits of soothing, oxygen-rich inhalations during labor. To complicate matters even more, what works for one mother doesn't always work for the next.

In short, there is still no single fail-proof formula for turning out perfect natural childbirths every time. For this reason, the Swiss training program for natural childbirth offers a wide range of safe breathing techniques, based on years of experience (and frustrations) with both the basic Read and Lamaze methods of childbirth preparation. During labor, it's up to the mother herself to choose those techniques which meet her individual needs.

For best results give yourself ample time to learn the various techniques at a leisurely pace by starting to practice in the second trimester of your pregnancy. Before going into these various techniques, let's look at the basics of breathing.

BREATHING FUNDAMENTALS

1. Breathing is an involuntary act which is automatically controlled by the respiratory center, a group of nerve cells within the medulla oblongata (the lowest part of the brain).

2. The respiratory center sends out rhythmic nerve impulses to the rib muscles and the diaphragm, causing them to contract and relax. This results in the three natural breathing movements:

    Breathing in (inhalation)
    Breathing out (exhalation)
    Breathing pause

3. No effort need be made to control inhalation, because the carbon dioxide content in the blood stimulates the respiratory center and breathing in takes place involuntarily. Therefore, inhalation should always be allowed to occur naturally, according to the rhythmic nerve impulses sent out by the respiratory center (see Figure 8-1). You can learn the three natural breathing movements by way of the simple sigh: Just sigh deeply and then wait until you feel a need for breath before inhaling. This slight pause between exhalation and inhalation is known as the "natural breathing pause."

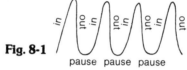

Fig. 8-1

pause   pause   pause

4. Any form of breathing that interferes with the natural three-beat rhythm, or in which breathing in is forced instead of allowed to occur involuntarily, is known as *controlled breathing.*

5. The three basic breathing levels are:

    a. *Deep (abdominal) breathing:* With one hand on your stomach, inhale slowly, drawing the air in toward your hand and trying to push up your hand (Figure 8-2). Inhaling at this level causes the diaphragm (the thin, arched breathing muscle separating the abdominal

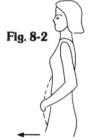

Fig. 8-2

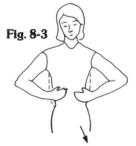

Fig. 8-3

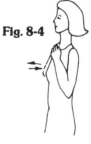

Fig. 8-4

and chest cavities) to sink down into its lowest position, increasing the size of the chest and allowing the
lungs to expand to full capacity.
  b. *Middle (intercostal) breathing:* With hands on ribs,
inhale slowly, drawing the air into your hands and
trying to spread them farther apart (Figure 8-3). At
this level the diaphragm does not swing down all the
way with each inhalation. Instead the intercostal (between the ribs) muscles are used to pull the ribs
farther apart, expanding the ribcage so that air can
rush into the lungs.
  c. *High (chest) breathing:* With shoulders relaxed and
one hand on your chest, just below the collarbone,
inhale toward your hand, causing chest to heave
(Figure 8-4). At this level the natural up and down
motion of the diaphragm is reduced even more and
only the upper part of the lungs expand. Such shallow
breathing should not be done for long, since it merely
ventilates the bronchial tubes (through which air
enters the lungs) but does not provide an adequate
supply of air in the alveoli, the tiny air sacs of the
lungs where the wastes in the blood are exchanged
for fresh oxygen.

A FEW WORDS OF CAUTION

Done repeatedly, controlled breathing (such as panting) can
cause hyperventilation, an imbalance in the levels of oxygen
and carbon dioxide in the body which results in an increase in
the alkalinity of the blood. When this occurs during pregnancy
or labor, the amount of oxygen in the blood reaching the fetus
is suddenly reduced and the mother becomes dizzy and feels
a prickling in her hands and feet. By quickly cupping her
hands over her face and breathing deeply, this condition is
easily remedied. Nevertheless, don't let it happen to you!

Done as described, the breathing exercises in this book
are not conducive to hyperventilation. So follow instructions
carefully and stick to the following common-sense rules:

1. Keep breathing lessons short—10 minutes is about right.
2. Limit yourself to practicing only one new breathing technique at a time, unless otherwise indicated.

3. Don't be tempted to skip any of the preliminary exercises, "cheat" on the full-deep-breathing follow-ups, or to rush from one exercise to the next or repeat the same exercise without first stopping to rest and breathe naturally in between.
4. Never jump straight up following a breathing exercise. Instead, allow yourself time to stimulate your slowed-down blood circulation by proceeding as follows:
    a. Move hands and feet in and out, up and down, and around in circles both clockwise and counterclockwise.
    b. Slowly roll over to one side, drawing up your knees along the floor, and take a deep satisfying breath. Close your eyes and relax, letting your breathing take care of itself, just as it does when you sleep.
    c. Now prop up on your lower arm and do some good lazy stretching: Stretch your upper arm, your neck, and your spine. Yawn several times if you can, as if awakening from a good, restful sleep.
    d. Sit up straight, draw another deep breath and open your eyes.
    e. Rise slowly in stages, kneeling and pausing to draw another deep breath before standing up—first on one foot and then on the other.

BREATHING IN BETWEEN CONTRACTIONS
Throughout labor there will be pauses in between contractions. Take advantage of these intervals to fill up on oxygen—for both you and your baby. Following every contraction, draw one or two "cleansing," full-deep breaths, letting yourself "collapse" and sink farther down into your bed as you exhale. Then let your breathing take care of itself, just as it does when you sleep, until the onset of your next contraction.

FULL-DEEP BREATHING

Full-deep breathing, which should be used repeatedly during pregnancy, labor, and for the rest of your life, is nothing more than a slow, smooth-flowing combination of deep (abdominal), middle (intercostal), and high (chest) breathing.

Usually full-deep breathing is done through the nose, but for those first two "cleansing" full-deep breaths following every contraction, exhale through your mouth while softly hissing, *sssss*, to make certain that all the air is expelled from your lungs and to cut down on the chances of hyperventilation occurring. For best results, practice the following exercise both ways: exhaling through your nose and through your mouth. Either way, always empty your lungs first by exhaling forcefully and then waiting until you feel a need to inhale before you begin.

Full-deep breathing exercise

Starting position:
Lie on your back with knees comfortably propped up by a rolled cushion, and if you like, place a pillow under your head as well.

Movements:
1. Inhale slowly and steadily, drawing the air in through your nose and down into your throat while experiencing a wave-like feeling of expansion, starting at your belly and spreading upward toward your midriff and chest.
2. Pause a moment to enjoy that special feeling of "fullness."
3. Exhale through the nose (or through the mouth while hissing *sssss*), exerting just a slight amount of force, and feel your body deflate and collapse in exactly the reverse order.

    Note: *Don't overdo it by inhaling forcefully beyond your natural breathing capacity or by practicing repeatedly. For beginners 2-3 full-deep breaths at a time are enough during pregnancy.*

Tip for beginners: *Breathing in slowly and deeply is easier the first few times if you practice while thinking of the French vowels "a" (pronounced "ah"), accented è (pronounced as the long "a" in "day"), and "I" (pronounced as the long "e" in "be"). Just close your eyes and inhale very slowly while letting the ring of these vowels resound, one by one, in your imagination. Better still, practice while listening to the slow soothing call of your husband or helper: "Ahhhhhhhh and Aayyyyyyy and eeeeeeeee and o-u-t o-u-t o-u-t." . . .*

GRADUATED BREATHING

Graduated breathing is a uniquely comfortable, airy type of breathing which sets the diaphragm into a light quivering motion, causes the pelvis to widen all around, and helps relax the pelvic floor muscles. This type of breathing can be detected, ever so slightly, in the lower back and along the pelvic floor. The breathing itself is slow, mild, and soundless, with the air being drawn in very gently through the nose and slightly upward into the nasopharynx (the upper part of the pharynx) as if slowly savoring (not sniffing) the scent of your favorite perfume. When this is done correctly, the nostrils remain perfectly still and it feels as if the air were being drawn in through them by an imaginary suction pump located in the middle of your head, midway between your ears.

By widening the pelvis all around, breathing in this manner actually makes more room for the contracting uterus, relieving it of outside pressure in the lower back and abdomen —just there where it usually hurts the most.

The first step in learning graduated breathing is to find your nasopharynx. One way of doing this is by adding the following once or twice to the usual deep-conscious relaxation text given on page 114. But first dab some Olbas oil or Vicks on your nostrils to help clear the nasal air passages.

Locating the nasopharynx while practicing deep-conscious relaxation

Text:
"Concentrate on the inside of your mouth— your oral cavity. Feel how v-a-s-t and hollow this cavity is." ... PAUSE ... "Now travel farther back into your throat until you come to the uvula, the little bob over the root of your tongue. Slip through under it, turn upwards and you enter another cavity, located right in the middle of your head, midway between your ears. You are in your nasopharynx. Feel your way carefully around

Fig. 8-5

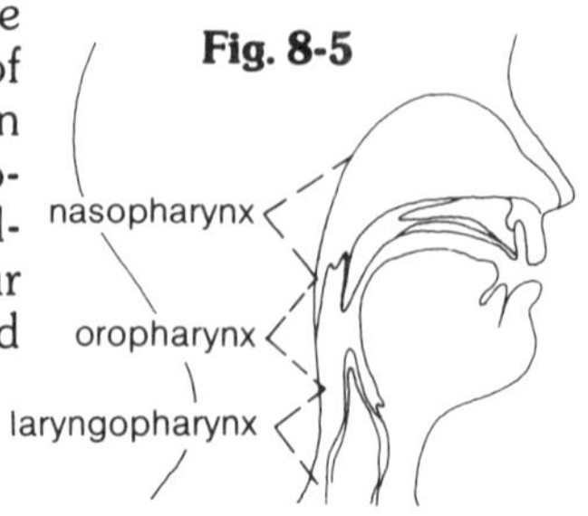

nasopharynx

oropharynx

laryngopharynx

and note how hollow this smaller cavity is."
. . . PAUSE . . . "Then very slowly and gently
breathe in the scent of the Olbas oil (or
Vicks), drawing it effortlessly in through
your nostrils and on toward this special
cavity in the middle of your head. Feel your
head slowly inflating, little by little, as it fills
with air.". . . PAUSE . . . "When you've inhaled
just enough to feel comfortably full, pause
briefly before letting your breath flow out
again, slowly and easily.". . . Pause again . . .
"Await the need-to-inhale before breathing
in slowly once more, into this hidden cavity
in the middle of your head. Don't force it.
Relax and make only the slightest effort to
guide the scent upwards. Relaxation and
graduated breathing go hand in hand. So let
g-o-o-o-o. Allow yourself to sink down and
be carried by the underlying bed (floor, etc.),
and continue to draw in and exhale the air in
this gentle, soothing manner, keeping in
time to your own natural breathing rhythm. . . ."

Tips for fathers: *To help your wife direct her breathing upward into her nasopharynx, place your hand lightly on the back of her head, midway between her ears, and encourage her to gently draw the air into your hand. If she is doing it right, you will actually be able to detect the faint movements of her breathing with your hand.*

THE DEEP, "RELAXING" SIGH

Once you've discovered the whereabouts of your nasopharynx you can go on to the next step—the slow, drawn-out sigh used at the start of the contraction to help you relax and thoroughly empty your lungs in preparation for the very slow inhalation of graduated breathing. To do it, draw a deep breath in through your nose, inflating your chest, and then let it out slowly and audibly through your mouth, carrying the tone down in a decrescendo for as long as you can (AHHHhhhhhh).

Put feeling into your sigh. It's a form of release. So let go and experience a wave of relaxation passing through your body as shoulders and chest "collapse," mouth and neck go loose, and pelvic floor eases.

You can take your time sighing because the start of a contraction is never very painful. If you use the first 8-10 seconds to sigh slowly and deeply, you will then be able to inhale more slowly, up and over the crest of the contraction wave, just at the time your contracting uterus is most sensitive to any outside pressure.

PROLONGING YOUR INHALATIONS
In all three forms of graduated breathing, the depth and length of your drawn-out inhalations depend directly on how far your lungs can expand. After all, the more air they can comfortably hold, the more you can comfortably inhale and the longer—and thus more effective—your graduated breathing will be.

Don't be discouraged if your inhalations seem too short at first. With diligent practice and some chest expansion exercises, not force, you can improve the natural breathing capacity of your lungs. So keep on practicing and timing yourself to note your own progress.

GRADUATED BREATHING: FIRST FORM
The first form of graduated breathing is the basic and simplest of the three forms. Inhaling is very slow and drawn out: it stops just short of the so-called bursting point when lungs are uncomfortably full and you feel choked by your own breath. If you inhale well within the limits of your own natural breathing capacity, you are able to pause at the top as you change over smoothly and comfortably from inhaling to exhaling, and you can control your exhalation instead of exhaling all the air at once out of a desperate need to empty your overfilled lungs. Exhaling is done in a very special step-by-step pattern, expelling the air in small measured doses, interjected with minute inhalations: OUT-in-OUT-in-OUT. . .

In Figure 8-6, the drawn out inhalation is shown as a wide curve stretching up and over the contraction wave and its intensity crest. The graduated "chopped-up" exhalation with its tiny inhalations is depicted here as a descending stairway of scalloped steps.

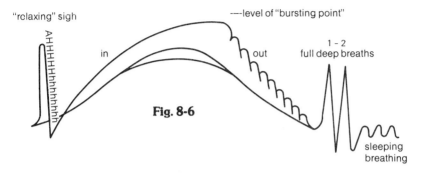

Fig. 8-6

Usually the first form of graduated breathing is suited for contractions lasting from 30-35 seconds, with a very small intensity crest.

Tip: *Study Figure 8-6 well and keep it in mind whenever you do the first form of graduated breathing. As you advance from one form to the next, always make a mental note of the relevant breathing illustration. You'll find that whichever form of graduated breathing you use, it helps to visualize the appropriate breathing pattern.*

Breathing Exercise for the First Form

Position:

The side-lying position is usually assumed during practice and labor, although all three forms of graduated breathing can also be done in the forward-leaning resting position (see page 169) or while kneeling on knees and elbows (see page 84). Whatever your position, close your eyes to help you relax and "tune in" to yourself. Remember that graduated breathing is a gentle, calming type of breathing. The more you let go-o-the easier and more effective it becomes. If your body is peaceful and relaxed, the air flows easily and gently into the nasopharynx, with only the slightest effort on your part—especially if you've dabbed your nostrils with some Olbas oil or Vicks VapoRub beforehand.

Note: *Don't make the common mistake of attempting to breathe into the nasopharynx with slightly parted lips. It cannot be done, so take special care to close your mouth after sighing the deep, relaxing sigh at the start of the contraction.*

Movements:
1. At the onset of the contraction, empty your lungs by sighing deeply with the relaxing sigh.
2. With lips closed, inhale slowly through your nose, *gently* drawing the air up into the middle of your head, and stop just before reaching your own individual bursting point.
3. Change over smoothly from inhaling to exhaling by pausing briefly at the peak.
4. Then exhale in the graduated step-by-step pattern: expel only a very small measure of air at a time and quickly retract a bit before exhaling another small measure of air. Continue in this pattern of expelling and retracting air—making sure that the amount exhaled always slightly exceeds the amount retracted—until all the air has been expelled from your lungs and the contraction has passed.
5. Follow up your graduated breathing by drawing one or two full, deep breaths (exhaling either through your nose or your mouth). Then relax and let your breathing take care of itself, just as it does when you sleep.

The best way to learn a new form of graduated breathing is to practice breathing over an imaginary contraction while listening to your husband (or helper) dictate the breathing movements in a low singsong tone of voice. The dictation for the first form (which should take about 35 seconds) is along these lines:

"Contraction begins! Draw a full, deep, breath i-n . . . let it out with a s-i-g-h: AHHHHhhhhhhh. . . . I-n-h-a-l-e v-e-r-y g-e-n-t-l-y up into the middle of your head, until your lungs are comfortably full . . . Pause at the top . . . Then: E-X-H-A-L-E . . . take-a-bit-back, O-U-T . . . and a-bit-in, O-U-T . . . and a-bit-in, O-U-T. . . . . End of contraction."

After practicing in this manner two or three times, try it again without the dictation. Instead your husband (or helper) should time the contraction out loud every few seconds while you breathe up and over the contraction wave according to your own natural breathing rhythm. In this way you can see for yourself just how long it takes you to sigh and to inhale, while breathing over a contraction with whichever form of graduated breathing is being practiced.

To check your breathing, the father or helper should lightly place his or her hand, palm down, over your tailbone. If you are doing it right the gentle up and down movements of your breathing can be easily detected with the hand. The movements of the simpler first form are somewhat less definable than those of the second and third.

When practicing by yourself, you can use this same hand-to-tailbone test to check your breathing.

Tip for fathers: *The timing and tone of the dictation is important. For the first form the dictation should take you approximately 35 seconds (not including "Contraction begins," and "Contraction ends"), with the first 8-10 seconds allowed for the very deep, relaxing sigh at the start. Speak slowly and quietly without any disconcerting stops and starts which might disturb your wife's relaxation. For best results read the text out loud to yourself once or twice and study the relevant breathing illustration before you begin.*

GRADUATED BREATHING: SECOND FORM

The second form of graduated breathing differs from the first in that the gradual inhalation is punctuated with several short exhalations in order to lengthen it and sustain the swelled-out state of the pelvic area over a longer intensity crest. Both the changeover pause at the top and the exhalation are the same as for the first form of graduated breathing.

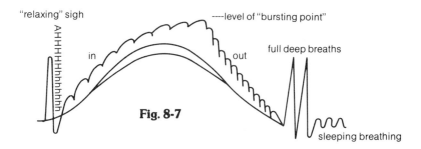

Fig. 8-7

In Figure 8-7 the inhalation pattern is illustrated as a mounting procession of small waves which gradually work their way up the contraction wave and over its crest—stopping just short of that now familiar bursting point. The graduated, step-by-step exhalation is again depicted as a descending stairway of scalloped formed steps.

The second form of graduated breathing is suited for contractions lasting anywhere from 40 to 60 seconds with an intensity crest of 20 to 30 seconds.

Breathing exercise for the second form

Starting position:
Same as for the first form.

Movements:
1. At the onset of the contraction, empty lungs by sighing deeply with the relaxing sigh.
2. Inhale by gently drawing a short breath of air into the nasopharynx and then

allowing a fraction of that air to escape
(IN-out-IN-out-IN . . .). Continue to draw
in and expel the air in this slow, graduating pattern—making sure that the
amount inhaled always exceeds the
amount expelled—until your lungs have
been comfortably filled.
3. Pause briefly at the top, until you feel the
   contraction losing some of its grip, and . . .
4. . . . begin exhaling in the usual step-by-
   step pattern.
5. As the contraction dies down, draw one
   or two full, deep breaths. Then relax and
   let your breathing fall effortlessly back
   into the passive, tranquil breathing used
   between contractions (sleeping-breathing).

Learning tips:
Since this form of graduated breathing can be used for contractions lasting 40-60 seconds (depending on the individual
needs of the mother), you should practice it both with and
without an accompanying text until you can do it effortlessly
for a full 60 seconds. Then keep practicing regularly (preferably at night just before falling sleep), since this is the breathing
technique you will be using most during labor.

Begin by breathing over an imaginary 45-second long
contraction while listening to your husband (or helper) dictate the breathing movements in a low, singsong tone of
voice. The dictation (which should take about 45 seconds) is
along these lines:

"Contraction begins! Draw a full deep breath
i-n . . . let it out with a s-i-g-h: AHHHHHhhhhhh." (8-10 seconds are up). "I-N-H-A-L-E
s-l-o-w-l-y—let-a-bit-out. I-N-H-A-L-E . . .
and a-bit-out. I-N-H-A-L-E . . . and a-bit-
out. I-N-H-A-L-E . . . and a-bit-out." Continue inhaling in this pattern until just before
your bursting point. Then, "C-h-a-n-g-e
o-v-e-r s-m-o-o-t-h-l-y to: E-X-H-A-L-E . . .
take-a-bit-back. O-U-T . . . and a-bit-in. O-U-T
. . . and-a-bit-in. O-U-T . . . and-a-bit-in.
O-U-T . . . end of contraction."

GRADUATED BREATHING: THIRD FORM

In the third form of graduated breathing, nostril or eventually open-mouth panting is added to the very slow, graduating inhalation, thereby enabling you to keep your pelvic area wide over a very long intensity crest. Once the contraction begins to let up, you can pass safely over into the graduated step-by-step exhalation.

The advantage of this breathing technique is that panting, which is very strenuous and which is conducive to hyperventilation, is limited to those few seconds when it is needed most to take the edge off a very long, intense contraction. By inhaling in the slow winding pattern at the start of the contraction and panting only later on, when the contraction is at the height of its intensity, you can cut down on your panting and save your strength without losing any of panting's effectiveness.

Nevertheless this more complex form of graduated breathing is not as relaxing and soothing as the others and should therefore be used *only* when the second form no longer seems adequate to keep you safely above your contractions.

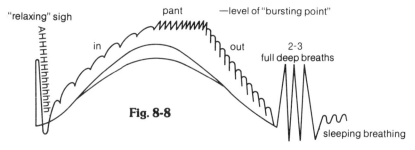

Fig. 8-8

In Figure 8-8 inhalation is illustrated this time as a somewhat shorter procession of waves that work their way up, but not over, the contraction and its intensity crest. Panting, with its rapid, two-beat rhythm, is depicted here as a zigzag of short, jagged angles making its way over the tip and latter half of the intensity crest. The graduated step-by-step exhalation is shown again as a descending stairway of scalloped steps.

The obvious prerequisite for learning the third form of

graduated breathing is knowing how to pant, both through the mouth and through the nose. You can do it either way, but as a rule nostril panting should be tried first, since panting through the open mouth is somewhat more superficial and more exhausting. It can also have a very annoying, drying effect on your mouth.

PRELIMINARY PANTING EXERCISES FOR THE THIRD FORM

Open-mouth panting

Starting position:
Sit at the edge of a chair with legs comfortably apart and feet flat on the floor. Keep back straight, with shoulders relaxed and torso tilted slightly forward. For learning purposes, place one hand lightly on your chest and try to push hand slightly up and down as you pant.

Movements:
1. Start by emptying your lungs with a good thorough sigh, inhaling through your nose and exhaling forcefully through your mouth.
2. As you finish exhaling, drop your chin, tilt head slightly down and thrust lower jaw out so that it protrudes noticeably in a somewhat unflattering (but nevertheless necessary) manner.
3. Keeping shoulders relaxed and tongue slack, resting limply in the middle of your mouth (encircled by air), start to pant lightly and rhythmically like a puppy, letting the air flow easily in and out through your open mouth. (You're doing it right if you can detect the slight rhythmic movements of your chest with your hand.) Continue to pant at an accelerated pace for 20 seconds; less if you feel uncomfortable.
4. Then end with a final exhalation.

5. Follow up by inhaling through your nose and blowing out through your mouth, 2 to 3 times.

Rest for two minutes before practicing panting through the nose:

Nostril panting

Starting position:
Same as for open-mouth panting.

Movements:
1. Sigh deeply, inhaling through the nose and exhaling very thoroughly through the mouth.
2. Purse lips lightly and . . .
3. . . . begin a light, rhythmic panting through your nose, gradually quickening your breathing rhythm as you go. Continue for 20 seconds; less if you feel uncomfortable.
4. End by exhaling through your mouth.
5. Follow up by inhaling through your nose and blowing out through your mouth, two to three times.

If you were able to pant both ways at an accelerated pace for a full 20 seconds, you can begin practicing the third form. If not, then repeat these two exercises once more and if necessary allow yourself a few more days time to practice before advancing to the third form of graduated breathing.

WARNING! Panting of any kind often results in hyperventilation and should therefore *not* **be practiced repeatedly during pregnancy.**

Breathing exercise for the third form

Position:
Use either the altered side lying position (see page 147) or any of the positions used for the other two forms, in which case you can ignore the head movements given below.

Movements:
1. At the onset of the contraction, empty your lungs by sighing very deeply with the deep, relaxing sigh.
2. Inhale slowly, drawing the air up into the middle of your head, in the same graduated pattern used for the second form but stopping well before reaching your own individual bursting point.
3. Roll head around, cradling it in your arm-pit, and begin panting rapidly and rhythmically, continuing until you feel the contraction weakening.
4. Then start the usual step-by-step exhalation and roll your head back to starting position.
5. Once the contraction has died down, draw two or three full, deep breaths and relax, letting your breathing fall back into a passive, tranquil breathing rhythm.

Tip for beginners: *The dictation for practicing the third form over a 60-second contraction is along these lines:*

"Contraction begins! Take a full, deep breath i-n . . . let it out with a S-I-G-H: AHHHH-hhhhhh." (8-10 seconds are up) "I-N-H-A-L-E s-l-o-w-l-y . . . let-a-bit-out. I-N-H-A-L-E . . . and a-bit-out. I-N-H-A-L-E . . . and a-bit-out. I-N-H-A-L-E . . . and a-bit-out. I-N-H-A-L-E . . . and a-bit-out. I-N-H-A-L-E, curl head quickly around and pant: tap, tap, tap, tap." (Father or helper claps hands in time to accelerated panting rhythm for 15 seconds.) "O-U-T . . . take-a-bit-in. O-U-T . . . and a-bit-in. O-U-T . . . and a-bit-in. O-U-T . . . and a-bit-in. O-U-T . . . and in. O-U-T. . . . End of contraction."

If you feel up to it, you can practice the third form two or three times during one session provided you take time out to rest quietly in between each "contraction."

Chapter Nine

JUST-IN-CASE BREATHING TECHNIQUES

During labor the contractions are usually strongest and the intervals between them are shortest at the very end of the first (dilation) stage and the very start of the second (expulsion) stage. This short, but relatively difficult period of labor is often referred to as "transition," although it is not a medical entity.

Usually the second or third form of graduated breathing is all a woman needs to keep her on top of her contractions at this time—but not always. If you should find yourself being overwhelmed by your contractions during transition despite your graduated breathing—or in the more likely event that you should experience an urge to push *before* being given the green light to do so—shift to low-panting.

LOW-PANTING

Low-panting is a unique form of intercostal breathing, practiced in an unnatural two-beat rhythm, which is very effective in combating pain and in counteracting the urge to push. It is based on the shallow, rapid panting taught by Dr. Fernand Lamaze of France to inhibit the sensations of pain during contractions. Because breathing on a shallow plane for long periods of time during labor has been harshly criticized (by many midwives and doctors) for limiting the amount of oxygen reaching the fetus and for exhausting the mother, the Swiss have replaced it with low-panting, which is easier to sustain and is done on a deeper plane. Nevertheless, low-panting should be used only as a last resort, when all three forms of graduated breathing fail to bring adequate relief or whenever you are instructed to resist your urge to push.*

*This is often the case when a mother feels the urge to push before her cervix (the uterine neck) is dilated enough to permit the passage of the baby's head. To push at such a time would be dangerous for both mother and child, as the soft fetal head would be pushed against the cervix instead of through it, possibly causing the cervix to tear.

HOW IT WORKS

The secret of low-panting's effectiveness for overcoming long, intense contractions lies in its ability to combat pain where it is first perceived: in the brain. When done at an accelerated pace, this form of controlled breathing requires so much concentration that the mother's brain is too preoccupied to perceive the nerve impulses sent from the contracting uterus as pain, in just the same way that the ball player might not notice a painful physical injury during an engrossing ball game.

In other words, it is not the breathing technique itself but the distraction it provides that makes low-panting work during a very intense contraction. On the other hand, when used to counteract the pushing reflex, low-panting works because the breathing rhythm itself makes it virtually impossible for the mother to retain enough air in her lungs to push with her diaphragm (as will be explained in Chapter 13).

HOW TO DO IT

Low-panting is done by inhaling a small quantity of air in through the mouth and down into the throat and then panting, low down, just beneath the breastbone, without letting any of the air flow in and out through the mouth as it does during high-level panting. The breathing is hollow, almost soundless, and is felt in the back of the throat. The slight movements of the breast cage and the fluttering diaphragm can be detected by lightly placing your fingertips on the very bottom (the xiphoid process) of your breastbone.

In a sense, low-panting is "playing ball" with the small quantity of air drawn into the windpipe (trachea). With mouth and tongue slack, throat relaxed, and the "trap" (epiglottis) open, the air is rhythmically "bounced" up—as if to inhale—and down—as if to exhale—without actually doing either, for at least 6 beats. Then, to ensure an adequate intake of oxygen, the used air is exchanged for fresh air, by a quick blowing out and breathing in.

LEARNING HOW

Before you try mastering the low-panting breathing technique, do the following preliminary exercises:

The quick, deep sigh

Whether used to overcome a difficult contraction or to counteract the urge to push, low-panting is effective only if you are able to catch the contraction at the very start—in time to quickly clear your lungs and begin low-panting before the contraction or the urge to push has gained the upper hand. This means that you don't have time to empty your lungs thoroughly with a slow, relaxing sigh (as you do by graduated breathing). Instead you must sigh quickly before you begin: inhaling through your nose and then blowing out the air through your mouth.

Reaching the required depth

With cupped hands, lightly place your fingertips on the very tip of your breastbone (xiphoid process; see Fig. 9-2). Vibrate the area gently to help you become more acutely aware of this part of your body. Then draw a quick breath in and sigh loudly, carrying the tone down in a decrescendo to the level of your fingertips. Unlike the relaxing sigh used for graduated breathing, this sigh does not linger on and is not used during actual labor. It serves only as a means of reaching the required depth necessary for panting low down.

The two-beat low-panting breathing rhythm

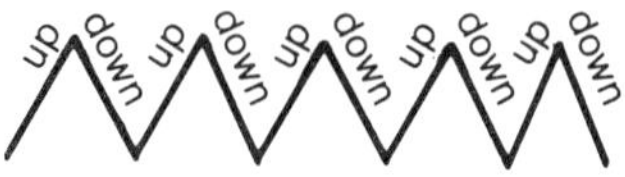

Fig. 9-1

Starting position:
Sit on a chair with legs spread comfortably apart and feet flat on the floor. Keep your back straight, with shoulders relaxed and tilt your torso slightly forward. To check the breathing movements, place fingertips of one hand lightly at the bottom of your breastbone and occasionally draw the back of the

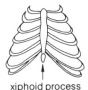

Fig. 9-2

xiphoid process
tip of sternum

other hand up to your mouth. To check the
the position of your head and jaw, practice in
front of a full-length mirror and lift your eyes,
not your head, from time to time to catch a
glimpse of yourself in the mirror.

Tip: *Low panting is easier with an open bra. It
also helps to do a few chest exercises (such as
elbow push-back and elbow circling) before
you begin.*

Movements:

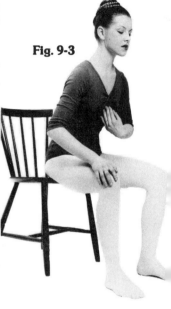

Fig. 9-3

1. Take a quick, but deep sigh to empty your
   lungs, breathing in through your nose and
   forcefully out through your mouth.
2. Drop your chin, lower your head, and
   thrust out your lower jaw so that it protrudes noticeably (Figure 9-3).
3. Keeping face, mouth, and throat loose,
   with the trap in the throat (epiglottis)
   open, suck in a spoonful of air through
   your mouth.
4. Thinking either "ha" or "ho," try to pant
   inwardly, low down beneath your breastbone, by rhythmically vibrating the air up
   and down without letting it escape through
   your open mouth. (You're doing it right if
   you can't feel the warmth of your breath
   on the back of your raised hand.)
5. When you feel the need, exhale and take
   1 or 2 full deep breaths, drawing the air
   in through your nose and out through
   your mouth.

Unless you feel dizzy at any point, you can repeat this exercise
twice, *providing you take a one-minute rest before each
repeat.* You should also take care to stop low-panting as soon
as you feel the need to catch your breath. Do not force
yourself to continue beyond your natural breathing capacity.

The low-panting breathing rhythm usually takes time to
master, so be patient. Practice it for several days. Then, when
you feel you're ready fot it, try learning how to punctuate it
with a quick exchange of air.

Exchanging the air with a SHHH-huuh

This is usually done by first vibrating the air up and down for 6 beats, then blowing out and quickly "vacuuming" in a fresh supply of air on the seventh. To make this rapid blowing-out and drawing-in of air easier, do it with a "SHHH-huuh" sound.

When this is done correctly, there is an even exchange of air and your tongue moves forward and upward toward the hard palate as you force out your breath on "SHHH," and then falls back to its original position (in the middle of your mouth) as you quickly vacuum in a spoonful of air on "huuh." To make certain that an even exchange of air takes place, do it 4-6 times in rapid succession and then stop abruptly. If you feel out of breath, then you were blowing out more than you were breathing in. Keep on trying until your "Shhh-huuh" is just right. Then combine it with low-panting as follows:

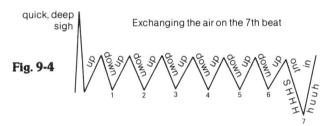

Fig. 9-4

quick, deep sigh

Exchanging the air on the 7th beat

The basic low-panting breathing technique

Starting position:
Same as for the two-beat low-panting breathing exercise.

Movements:
1. Take a quick, deep sigh, breathing in through the nose and blowing out through the mouth.
2. Drop the chin, lower the head, and thrust out the lower jaw.
3. Suck in a spoonful of air and pant rhythmically low down beneath your breastbone for 6 beats.

4. On the seventh beat push out the air (with "SHHH") and quickly draw in a fresh spoonful of air (with "huuh"). When this is done correctly, the warmth of the expelled breath can be felt on the back of your hand if you put it up to your mouth.
5. Continue in this pattern, low-panting and exchanging the air with a quick "SHHH-huuh" on every seventh beat for 30-40 seconds, eventually working up to 60. (Once you are able to do it for a full minute try doing it at an accelerated pace, gradually quickening your rhythm to match the mounting intensity of an imaginary contraction and then slowing down again as the contraction dies down.)
6. When you feel the need, end on an exhale and follow up with one or two full deep breaths, drawing the air in through your nose and forcefully out through your mouth.
7. Rest for two minutes before repeating this exercise. For beginners, practicing two or three times is enough.

Tip: *When practicing, you'll find it helps to clap your hands in time to your breathing rhythm, doing: tap-tap-tap-tap-tap-tap- SHHH-huuh; especially when trying to do it at an accelerated rate.*

Note: *For most women, exchanging the air on the seventh beat is just right, but not for all. Some prefer to do it, say, on the eleventh beat; this works just as well, as long as the woman feels comfortable and doesn't falter in her rhythm.*

LOW-PANTING VARIATIONS

LOW-PANTING ON AN AIR CUSHION

Some women complain of a slight shortness of breath while panting low down. If this is your problem, try retaining a small reserve of air in the lower part of your lungs as you low-pant. You can do this by first "vacuuming" in (as if with a suction pump) a small quantity of air, through your nose and down into your lungs, and low-panting on top of that. Whenever you're ready to exchange the air (with a quick "SHHH-huuh") take care to expel only the usual spoonful of air, not to empty your lungs of your air cushion.

"SNIFFLING"

As its name suggests, this somewhat simpler form of low-panting is done through the nose instead of the mouth, by panting lightly and rhythmically in the lower part of the nostrils, as if sniffling very gently. Just in case you should have to resort to low-panting to breathe over a few, long, intense contractions at the end of the first stage, you may find it more comfortable to switch to sniffling from time to time, as this form of low-panting is less strenuous and has no drying side effect.

Unlike other forms of low-panting, sniffling causes the ribcage to expand at the sides and the breathing, which is light and almost soundless, can be easily detected at the nostrils if you draw the back of your hand up in front of your nose.

Note: *Unless sniffling is used in combination with openmouth panting (described later), it's best not to use it to overcome a pushing contraction, as there is always the possibility that you will hold your breath when your mouth is closed.*

Sniffling exercise

Starting position:
Same as for open-mouth low-panting except that hands are placed on the sides of the ribs. Occasionally the back of one hand is drawn up to the nostrils to check if the gentle in-and-out flow of air can be detected.

Movements:
1. Take a quick, deep sigh.
2. Gently purse your lips.
3. Inhale a spoonful of air toward your hand and gently vibrate it rhythmically up and down for 6 beats, or for as long as

you comfortably can. (You are doing it right if you feel slight rhythmic movements under your hands.)

4. On the seventh beat (or later) open your lips and let out your breath while *whispering* a quick, explosive "poo."
5. Quickly purse your lips and start again from step 3.
6. Continue in this pattern of rhythmically sniffling and exchanging the air with "poo" for 30-40 seconds before slowing down and ending with a final prolonged "poooo."
7. Follow up by drawing one to two full, deep breaths (in through the nose and out through the mouth) and then resting for at least one full minute.
8. Repeat two or three times.

Practice "sniffling" for several days. Then try doing combined low-panting.

COMBINED LOW-PANTING

During labor, if you should need to low-pant over a very long intense contraction, or if you have to counteract a premature urge to push, it helps to sandwich open-mouth low-panting between two layers of the somewhat simpler sniffling. In this way you can start and end with sniffling and low-pant through your mouth only in the middle, just when your contraction is at its peak. This pattern is illustrated in Figure 9-5.

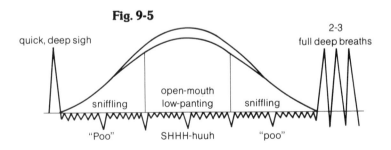

Fig. 9-5

quick, deep sigh

2-3 full deep breaths

sniffling   open-mouth low-panting   sniffling

"Poo"   SHHH-huuh   "poo"

Combined low-panting exercise

Position:
Same as for open-mouth low-panting, except that one hand rests on one side of your rib-cage (to check your sniffling) and the fingertips of the other hand rest lightly on the tip of your breastbone (to check your open-mouth low-panting).

Tip: *While panting through your mouth, draw the hand that rests on the side of your rib-cage up in front of your mouth to check whether or not any of the air is escaping.*

Movements:
1. Take a quick, deep sigh.
2. Purse lips and . . .
3. . . . quickly draw a spoonful of air in through your nose and begin sniffling (with an occasional "poo") at an accelerated pace.
4. As the contraction mounts in intensity, smoothly but quickly switch to open-mouth low-panting by opening your mouth to expel the air with a short, explosive "poo," then quickly sucking in a fresh spoonful of air through your mouth, and thrusting out your lower jaw.
5. Low-pant through your mouth, accelerating your rhythm as the contraction grows stronger and exchanging the air with "Shhh-huuh" on every seventh beat (or later).
6. As the contraction begins to ease, reduce the pace of your low-panting and revert smoothly but quickly to sniffling. This changeover is done by exhaling through your mouth on "Shhh" and then quickly pursing your lips and inhaling a fresh spoonful of air through your nose.

7. Continue sniffling, gradually slowing down your tempo as the contraction dies down. End by expelling the air with a final, forceful "pooo."
8. Once the contraction has passed, relax and draw a full deep breath in through your nose and out through your mouth two or three times.
9. Relax for at least one minute before repeating this exercise. If you feel up to it you can practice combined low-panting two to three times, always stopping to rest in between.

ALTERNATE POSITIONS

After learning the rudiments of low-panting, practice it in all of the following positions:

LEANING-BACK POSITION

Rest in a half-lying position with torso supported at a 45-degree angle as if reclining in a deck chair. Knees are spread hip-width apart and bent at the knees. Eyes are wide open. (It helps to place fingertips at the very tip of your breastbone.) See Figure 9-6.

It is easier to pant sitting up than lying down. However, you should use this leaning-back position only when low-panting to counteract the urge to push; not to overcome a very hard, long contraction during transition. Leaning back during such a contraction would be adding unnecessary pressure on the nerves in your lower back.

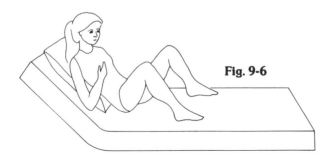

Fig. 9-6

ALTERED SIDE-LYING POSITION

You may never feel the need to use low-panting during the first stage of labor, but just in case you do you'll find it much more relaxing and comfortable if you remain lying in the side-lying position but with your head resting on your arm, at the wrist, instead of on the pillow (see Figure 9-7). At the onset of the contraction, draw a deep breath and roll your head around, cradling your forehead in your arm (as shown in Figure 9-8). In this position your breast cage is slightly elevated and free, enabling you to sigh and low-pant in greater comfort. At the conclusion of the contraction just roll your head around to starting position (on the back of your wrist) and draw one or two full, deep breaths, always drawing the air in through your nose and out through your mouth.

Fig. 9-7

Fig. 9-8

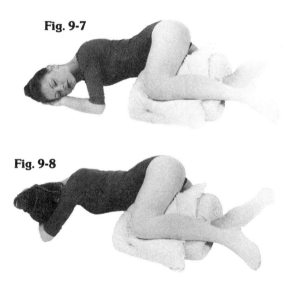

This slightly altered side-lying position is also suitable for panting while doing the third form of graduated breathing.

Note: *Remove watch and eyeglasses before settling down in this position.*

ON ALL FOURS

Probably the best way to low-pant over a contraction would be to kneel down on all fours. Unfortunately, this cannot always be done at the hospital, where it is still an unusual sight in many parts of the modern world, and where the use of fetal monitors and I.V's could make getting into this position cumbersome. Nevertheless, you should practice low-panting on all fours every now and then, since most women find it easier to learn in this position, possibly because the lower jaw droops naturally when relaxed and the chest is free.

Kneel on hands and knees with hands at right angles to shoulders and knees at right angles to hips (see Figure 9-9). Keep spine and head aligned and swallow hard before you begin in order to avoid drooling.

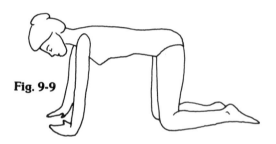

Fig. 9-9

Chapter Ten

UNDERSTANDING THE EXPULSION (SECOND) STAGE OF LABOR

Once the cervix is fully dilated and you are given the okay to push, the expulsion stage—the most agreeable and satisfying phase of the whole labor—is well underway. Now, at last, the door to your womb is wide open and your baby is ready to embark on one of life's most perilous journeys—the passage through the narrow birth canal. Only you, the mother, can ease and speed him on his way in the gentlest and safest way known to man.

PHYSIOLOGY OF SECOND-STAGE LABOR

At the start of each pushing contraction the thicker muscular portion of the uterus (the upper segment) is drawn back and shortened, thereby thickening the upper border (the fundus) and transforming it into a thick, forceful plunger which thrusts the baby downward. (See Figure 10-1.) The forceful down-thrust of the uterus is comparable to a weight of at least 55 pounds, yet it alone is not enough to propel the baby out—you have to help. Fortunately nature is on your side. The contractions of second-stage labor are almost always marked by an irresistible urge to push, very similar to the urge to

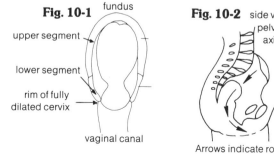

Fig. 10-1
fundus
upper segment
lower segment
rim of fully dilated cervix
vaginal canal

Fig. 10-2 side view of the bony pelvis and its axis (or curve)

Arrows indicate route baby travels

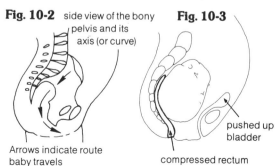

Fig. 10-3
pushed up bladder
compressed rectum

empty the bowels, only much stronger. These contractions are usually longer and stronger than those of the first stage. Nevertheless, they are not painful. On the contrary, following your urge to push feels good—if you know how.

When mother and uterus join forces, the baby is pushed steadily farther along through the narrow, winding birth canal (Figure 10-2) with each contraction, and slips back slightly as the contraction subsides. In his descent the baby travels downward toward his mother's lower spine, before hitting bottom (the inside of her pelvic floor) and twisting his way around the natural curve of her pelvis and forward toward the front.

To make more room for himself on his way the baby compresses his mother's rectum; thus the pushing reflex (Figure 10-3) pushes her bladder up and eventually pushes back her coccyx (temporarily) as he passes by the tail end of her spine. Somewhere along the way the amniotic sac of waters, which warmed and protected him from jolts and jars, will break or be ruptured manually, making his journey just that much more difficult.

Fortunately, there are no sensory nerves in the cervix or in the upper part of the vagina, and the nerves of the pelvic floor are usually temporarily numbed when the baby presses against them, slowing down their blood supply and stretching the perineum. In fact, if you should tear or be cut (episiotomy) at this point you might not even notice it.* Only as the baby "crowns"† and your work is almost done is there a chance of your experiencing a light tingling sensation at and around the vaginal outlet (similar to the prickling felt when your leg falls asleep) or possibly a feeling of "splitting open" (as when passing a very hard bowel movement). These minor discomforts pass within seconds, unless you mistakenly react by tightening up your pelvic floor and keeping your baby back— a very unlikely reaction for a "prepared" mother.

Once you've come this far you'll be far too excited and busy watching your baby being born to notice anything else.

---

*Sometimes a little Novocain is injected into the mother's perineum for the episiotomy.
†When the crown of the baby's head can be seen at the outlet with the vulva bulging over it.

MOTHER'S ROLE DURING THE SECOND STAGE

When your baby is being forced down the narrow birth canal, you can help him come through safely and quickly by keeping alert, following orders, and pushing effectively in the right direction at just the right time. In fact, the more effective your push, the sooner your baby will be born. Don't confuse pushing hard with pushing effectively. A good satisfying push that gets results and affords relief takes less energy than a frantic one in the wrong direction. It is more a matter of timing, technique, and good muscle tone than physical strength.

TIMING

Because your uterus needs part of each contraction to pull back its upper segment and thicken at the top (the fundus) before it can bear down, you have ample time at the start of each expulsive contraction to catch and hold a bolster of air in your lungs and then get into position *before* starting to push. Bearing down ahead of your uterus would be merely a waste of energy. You simply cannot do it alone. Figure 10-4 is a diagram illustrating the coordinating of your push with the downthrust of the uterus.

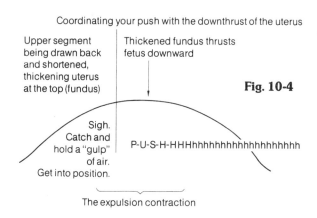

Coordinating your push with the downthrust of the uterus

Upper segment being drawn back and shortened, thickening uterus at the top (fundus)

Thickened fundus thrusts fetus downward

Fig. 10-4

Sigh. Catch and hold a "gulp" of air. Get into position.

P-U-S-H-HHHhhhhhhhhhhhhhhhhhhhhh

The expulsion contraction

TECHNIQUE

Unless you plan to give birth squatting down (the way your distant ancestors did), you need special, step-by-step training in the intricate art of effective pushing. Otherwise, following your natural urge to push while lying on your back with your legs drawn up and spread apart can be tricky: If you push as if to empty your bowels you might instinctively tighten up your pelvic floor muscles as you feel both vaginal and anal outlets opening up—acting out of a mistaken (but correctable) reflex to keep yourself from possibly defecating in this awkward, vulnerable position. (After all, tightening the pelvic floor is obviously not the normal reaction to pushing during elimination.) On the other hand, if you push as if to forcefully empty your bladder, your pelvic floor muscles will relax but so will your abdominal wall, allowing the force of your push to be channeled into your belly instead of in the direction of the curved birth passage. To avoid making these or other errors at a time when every second counts, learn how to reinforce the explosive efforts of your uterus and add force and direction to your own push by:

1. *Pushing steadily against the top of your uterus with your diaphragm.* By quickly filling your lungs with a bolster of air, you bring your diaphragm to sink down in the center and push against the fundus of your uterus, thereby adding to the force of its downthrust. Since you can't keep your diaphragm fixed in this lowered position without air in your lungs, you need to be able to hold your breath for as long as you comfortably can while you push. Every time you do stop to catch your breath, your diaphragm swings back up into its arched position, momentarily interrupting your push. With practice you should be able to push during a contraction without stopping more than three times to catch a fresh gulp of air.
2. *Bracing your abdominal muscles by curling head and shoulders forward.* If you forget to do this—or if your abdominal wall is lax due to poor muscle tone—some of the force being exerted by your diaphragm and your uterus to push the baby downward toward the small of your back and tailbone will be lost as the abdominal wall "gives."
3. *Pushing in the right direction.* Instead of pushing uselessly

up into your head or merely puffing out your belly, aim your push carefully in the direction of the birth canal. Remember that because of the natural curve of the pelvic canal the baby cannot descend straight down in front.

Instead he travels . . . farther *down* into his mother's pelvis, heading toward her lower back (Figure 10-5); turns around the bend of her pelvis (internal rotation) as he meets the resistance of her pelvic floor muscles (Figure 10-6); and continues *forward* along her pelvic floor and out to his "crowning" (Figure 10-7).

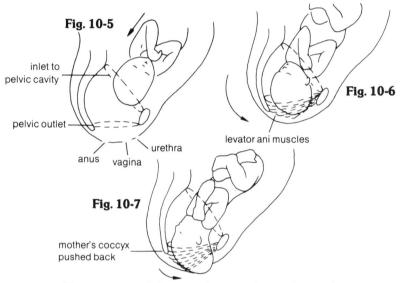

Fig. 10-5

inlet to
pelvic cavity

pelvic outlet

anus   vagina   urethra

Fig. 10-6

levator ani muscles

Fig. 10-7

mother's coccyx
pushed back

You can speed him on his way by pushing: down, under your ribs, toward your lower back, and then forward (and slightly uphill if you're lying on your back) around to the front of your pelvic floor (Figure 10-8).

4. Consciously relaxing buttocks and pelvic outlets as you push forward along the pelvic floor.

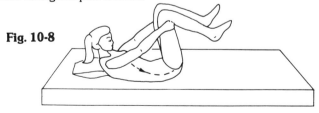

Fig. 10-8

GOOD MUSCLE TONE

Good muscle tone in the abdominal wall is vital to your push because it helps compress the uterus downward through the pelvis. To give you a good idea of just how this works, consider the basic mechanics of an ordinary syringe (see Figure 10-9). In order to eject the serum that is in the hollow barrel, two things are necessary: the force exerted from above by the plunger as it pushes down, and the counter-pressure exerted by the walls of the barrel. If the barrel should "give" by expanding sideways, the serum would flow in all directions, instead of being completely ejected downward into the hollow needle at the bottom.

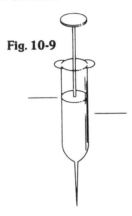

Fig. 10-9

The downward pressure exerted by the plunger is comparable to the pressure exerted by the mother's diaphragm and the fundus of the uterus as they push down to expel the baby. The counter-pressure exerted by the firm "walls" of the barrel are comparable to the counter-pressure exerted by the mother's braced abdominal wall.

Chapter Eleven
PERFECTING YOUR PUSH

The best and easiest way to learn how to push effectively during labor is by practicing the "natural way"—while moving your bowels. Of course, during childbirth itself you will have to direct your push a little bit farther forward, past the anus to the vagina. But the general route is basically the same, and once you've reached and pushed open the anus, the rest is easy.

Unfortunately, we in the West have grown so out of touch with nature that most of us simply don't know how to push effectively without straining hard during the normal everyday act of elimination—let alone during childbirth! Even our toilet seats are constructed all wrong: they should be lower to allow for a squatting position.* To compensate for this fault, you should practice your push with your feet raised a few inches off the floor, placed on footstools, shoeboxes, or any other handy objects of similar height. But first do all of the following:

PRELIMINARY EXERCISES FOR LEARNING HOW TO PUSH

Holding in your breath

Position:
Sit on the edge of a chair with knees spread hip-width apart and feet set firmly on the floor. Lean slightly forward, keeping your back, neck, and head aligned and rest your hands on your thighs just above your knees.

Movements:
1. Roll your head back, stretching your neck, and quickly catch a "gulp" of air in

---

*To correct this, many of the newer toilets are being constructed with a lower seat and a floor that is built on an incline.

through your mouth. Make sure the amount inhaled is not uncomfortable.

2. Quickly hold and block the air by pursing your lips, tucking your chin in, and consciously closing the "trap" (the epiglottis) in the throat.

3. Wait quietly, with chest, shoulders, and neck relaxed. (To make sure they are, gracefully sway shoulders to and fro while holding in your breath.)

4. When you feel uncomfortable, roll your head back and let your breath out with a quick but explosive "ahh."

5. Follow up with two full, deep breaths.

Note: *Time yourself while practicing. You need to work up to 40 seconds in order to be able comfortably to hold your breath and push for 10 seconds straight during a real contraction, before stopping to catch a fresh gulp of air. Improving your ability to hold your breath takes practice and patience but it can be done, so keep on trying.*

Candle blowing

Starting position:
Rest on the floor or mat in a half-lying position, with elbows and lower arms tucked under for support, fingers pointing forward. Keep legs comfortably apart and stretched out loosely, with knees slightly bent and feet on the floor.

Movements:
1. Imagine a cluster of candles between your legs and try to blow them out one by one with several quick, short blows and then one long-lasting one (Figure 11-1).

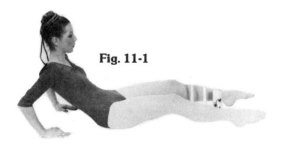

Fig. 11-1

As you blow, note what physical sensations you perceive in your body. When this is done properly, you should feel a definite tug beneath your ribs just as you should when you push during delivery.

Practicing the "natural way"

Starting position:
Sit on the toilet seat with feet set firmly on a raised surface (of approximately 6 inches) and knees spread comfortably apart. Lean forward and rest your lower arms on your thighs, with elbows slightly bent.

Movements:
1. Sigh deeply.
2. Throw head back and catch a gulp of air.
3. Hold and block the air by pursing lips and tucking chin in to help shut the epiglottis.
4. While lifting elbows out at the sides, push steadily in the following direction: *downward,* under the ribs; *downward,* toward the small of the back and the tailbone; and *forward,* to the anus and the vagina, opening them up w-i-d-e.
5. When you feel the need, roll your head back and expel the air while whispering a quick, explosive "ahhh."

Caution: *When practicing during elimination take care not to strain hard. Even when you practice pushing in any of the positions used during second stage.labor, don't push full force, but only enough for you to be aware of a slight pull beneath your ribs and a gentle widening of your anal and vaginal outlets. Although it is very unlikely that the bag of waters surrounding your baby could rupture or leak from the force of your push, it is not altogether impossible. Besides, straining hard could very well encourage hemorrhoids or aggravate existing ones.*

Common mistakes:

1. *Inhaling too much air.* When this happens, you feel "choked" by your own breath and need to exhale quickly.

2. *Straining into your head.* If you face is all twisted and red, with puffed-up cheeks and popped-out veins, you are doing one or both of two things:

   a. Blocking the air with your lips alone instead of closing the "trap" in your throat and tucking your chin in to help keep it shut. When this happens you naturally strain into your head instead of holding the compressed air down against the diaphragm.

   b. Straining too hard because your push is aimed in the wrong direction—forward into your belly, causing it to swell—instead of keeping your abdominal muscles braced. To correct this, try thinking of the route your baby is taking as you push: downward toward the small of your back and tailbone, and then forward to the front of your pelvic floor.

3. *Pressing elbows against ribs* as you push instead of holding them up and out at the sides in order to brace your rib muscles. This is a seemingly small error that makes a big difference. To avoid this common mistake, make it a point to practice pushing with elbows up and out until it becomes a habit.

PUSHING POSITIONS

Once you've perfected your push you can take it a step farther and practice pushing in the various positions actually assumed during delivery.

The leaning-back sitting position

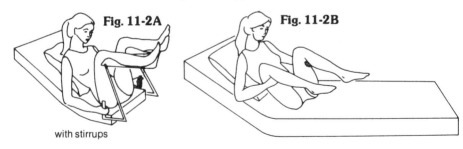

Fig. 11-2A

with stirrups

Fig. 11-2B

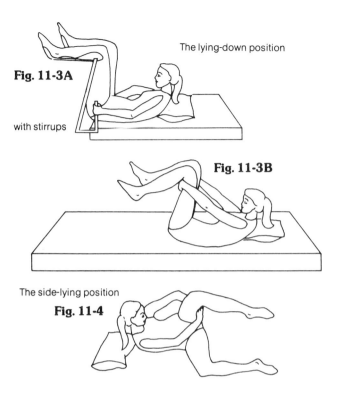

Fig. 11-3A
with stirrups

The lying-down position

Fig. 11-3B

The side-lying position
Fig. 11-4

As you can see from the illustrated pushing positions, stirrups may or may not be used when either the lying-down or the leaning-back sitting position is assumed. When stirrups are not used the mother has to hold her thighs in place and use her legs for leverage to pull head and shoulders up into a comfortable pushing position. When stirrups are used the mother's legs are first put up into the stirrups and then the lower end of her bed (which is actually a delivery table) is removed so that her buttocks rest on the very edge of the "broken" delivery table. This allows the attending physician or midwife easier access to her pelvic floor and to the emerging baby and eliminates the need for the mother to hold her legs in place or to use her legs to pull herself up into position. Instead, she can use the hand grips at the sides of the delivery table.

If you are scheduled to give birth in a hospital where stirrups are the accepted rule, skip the exercise for pushing without them. On the other hand, if you are planning to give birth without stirrups, practice pushing both ways, since you cannot be certain that you will not ultimately need stirrups in unforeseen complications. In any case, practice pushing in the side-lying position as well, since you may be asked to push on your side, especially if the position of the baby needs to be corrected.

Exercise for pushing without stirrups

Starting position:
Lie flat on the floor with your knees bent, hip-width apart and your hands resting on your chest. Keep your eyes open.

Movements:
1. At the onset of the "contraction," sigh deeply—in through the nose and out through the mouth.
2. Catch a quick gulp of air.
3. Hold and block air, pursing lips and tucking chin in.
4. Draw right knee up and hook your wrist under it (this is much easier than grasping behind your thighs).
5. Do the same with left arm and left knee.
6. Pull arms, head, and shoulders up by drawing legs forward until knees are parallel to hips. Don't force it and don't rush. Relax and let your legs work to pull you up into a comfortable position (see Figure 11-3b).
7. As head curls forward, lift elbows out at the sides and push in the following direction: under your ribs, toward the small of your back and your tailbone, and forward along your pelvic floor, past the anus to the vagina, opening them up w-i-d-e.

8. When you feel the need to exhale, roll your head back, straightening your neck, and let the air rush out through your open mouth while uttering a soft but explosive "ahh." (While you are letting your breath out, the downward pressure of the diaphragm is momentarily lifted. Be careful not to lose the counterpressure of your braced abdominal wall as well by letting go of your legs and lowering your head, shoulders, and elbows.)

9. Quickly catch a fresh gulp of air. Block and hold as you curl head forward and p-u-s-h for as long as you can comfortably hold your breath (the longer the better).

10. Repeat steps 8 and 9.

11. End by dropping elbows and rolling head and shoulders back down on the floor. Release your right leg with control, gently returning it to its original starting position, with knee bent and foot flat on the floor. Then do the same with your left arm and leg. (During practice and during labor, never release both legs at once allowing them to flop down on the underlying surface.)

12. Follow up with two full, deep breaths.

13. Do 2-3 times, pausing to rest in between.

Note: *Practice pushing often during pregnancy until the movements become automatic and fluid.*

Exercise for pushing with stirrups

Starting position:
Lie on the floor directly in front of a well upholstered armchair or sofa, with your knees drawn up, hip-width apart and calves resting on the seat of the armchair or sofa. Place your hands on your chest and keep your eyes open.

Tip: *If someone holds onto the back of the armchair, you can use the front legs of the armchair as substitute hand grips; otherwise pull head and shoulders up by grasping low down behind your thighs with your hands.*

Movements:
1. Sigh deeply at the onset of the "contraction."
2. Catch a quick gulp of air.
3. Hold and block the air, closing your mouth and tucking chin in.
4. Grasp the lower ends of your substitute hand grips or grasp behind your thighs as illustrated in Figure 11-5a.
5. Pull on your "hand grips" or on your thighs and spread elbows outward at the sides to pull head and shoulders up (Figure 11-5b), and . . .

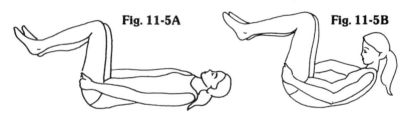

Fig. 11-5A   Fig. 11-5B

6. . . . push steadily (for as long as you can hold down the air) in the following direction: under the ribs, toward the small of the back and the tailbone, and forward to the anus and the vagina, opening them up w-i-d-e.
7. When you feel the need, roll head back and let your breath out with a short, explosive "Ahh." (Be careful not to let go of the "hand grips" or to lower your head and shoulders!)
8. Catch and hold a fresh gulp of air; curl head forward, and . . .
9. . . . push continuously for as long as you can comfortably hold your breath.

10. Repeat steps 7, 8, and 9.
11. End by returning head and shoulders to their original resting position and drawing hands back, well out of the sterile field.
12. Follow up with two full, deep breaths.
13. Repeat 1-2 times, allowing yourself to rest in between each "contraction."

Note: *While stirrups that are well adjusted have been known to add to the mother's comfort, the opposite is true of stirrups that are set too far apart, too high, or too low for comfort. Fortunately, stirrups are adjustable. So if you should find them uncomfortable, speak up and ask the nurse to please adjust them to fit your individual anatomy.*

Exercise for pushing in the (right) side-lying position

Starting position:
Lie on your right side, with arms drawn up in front and bent at the elbows so that hands are at eye level. Keep your legs together, bent at the knees and drawn up so that your thighs are at right angles to your hips (Figure 11-6a).

Movements:
1. At the onset of the "contraction," sigh deeply.
2. Catch and hold a quick gulp of air as you . . .

Fig. 11-6A

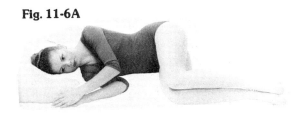

3. ... slowly draw your upper (left) thigh toward your chest and grasp it with your upper (left) arm (Figure 11-6b).
4. Remaining on your right hip, turn slightly toward the left (without rolling over on your back) and hook your lower (right) arm under your raised thigh. Then, in one smooth continuous motion draw raised leg forward (away from torso) letting it pull head and shoulders up and bend elbows out at the sides (see Figure 11-6c), forming a little opening through which to watch for your baby as you ...
5. ... p-u-s-h: down, toward the small of your back and the tail end of your spine, and around to the front of your pelvic floor.

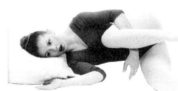

Fig. 11-6B

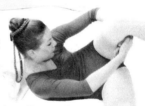

Fig. 11-6C

6. When you feel the need, roll your head back and let out your breath with a quick, explosive "ahh."
7. Catch another quick gulp of air. Hold and block air, curling head forward, and push for as long as you can before stopping for breath.
8. Repeat steps 6 and 7.
9. End by letting your breath out with the usual "ahh" and then slowly turn back down on your right side and return to starting position.

INTERRUPTING YOUR PUSH ON COMMAND

"Crowning" is the term used to describe that very special moment when the tip of your baby's head can be seen peeking through the vaginal outlet. Soon you can catch a glimpse of his face, but first your doctor or midwife must go about the delicate task of working the head out slowly.

Pushing now could be a mistake, since you need to go easy on the baby's fragile head and on your perineum which is stretched extremely thin and could easily tear. The doctor or midwife will guide you. At just the right moment—during crowning and when the baby is coming too quickly—you will be given a command to "stop pushing." When this happens, you must be able instantly to stop your push short by rolling your head and shoulders back down on the table, dropping your elbows (without letting go of thighs or hand grips), throwing back your head, and panting quickly through your open mouth—until you are told to push or until the contraction ends.

The ability to respond in a flash and stop pushing right in the middle of a contraction is no small feat. The pushing reflex usually is extremely strong. Don't underestimate it! Counteracting your urge to push during a contraction takes training. So practice often, preferably with your husband acting as doctor and coach by calling out the shots in turn: "Contraction begins. Sigh; gulp; hold and block; get into position and p-u-s-h-h-h-h——stop pushing——p-u-s-h-h-h-h——stop pushing——p-u-s-h-h-h-h. Contraction is over."

For best results, time yourselves, allowing between 50 and 70 seconds for each pushing contraction, with the first few seconds being used to get ready (sigh, gulp, block, and assume position).

Although these little rehearsals can be fun, they are not to be taken lightly. When it's for real, your ability to respond immediately upon command, and to make the most out of every pushing contraction, will determine to a great extent how long your baby's stay in the narrow birth canal will be.

III.
PRACTICAL
APPLICATION

Chapter Twelve

MANAGING LABOR

THE ONSET OF LABOR: WHAT NOW?

Don't rush to the hospital or climb into bed with those first few contractions, especially if this is your first baby. Continue doing whatever you were doing, or else go for a walk with your husband, preferably up and down a hilly street. Walking around helps move the baby farther down into the pelvic basin and is likely to intensify your contractions. Which is *just* what you want to do at this point.

Sometimes labor is preceded by hours of lazy, mild contractions. When such a contraction becomes too noticeable to be comfortably ignored, bend forward from the waist and lean over anything suitable that is handy: the kitchen sink, the office typewriter, or if you're outdoors, a tree trunk or lamp post, and until the contraction subsides, breathe quietly; using either full, deep breathing, or one of the first two forms of graduated breathing. Your position is important. (See Figures 12-1 and 12-2.) When you round your back, the pelvic inlet widens and the spine moves slightly backward, reducing pressure (which is easily translated into pain) on the sacral nerves.

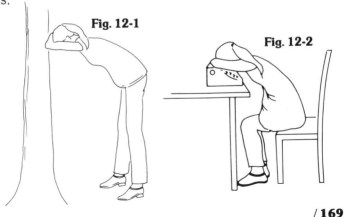

Fig. 12-1

Fig. 12-2

Rounding your back is a simple, common-sense measure which can make your entire labor far more comfortable, so keep it in mind both at home and at the hospital. Don't sit up and lean back in a bed or on a chair, and don't lie on your back until you feel the urge to push.

Before you leave for the hospital there are a number of other common-sense measures which you may like to try:

SELF-MASSAGE
For contractions that are felt more strongly in the lower back, combine your breathing (either full, deep breathing or the first two forms of graduated breathing) with a self-massage. Use either one or both of the following massages:

The push-back self-massage
Starting position:
Stand with feet slightly apart, knees well bent, and back leaning against a wall that is approximately an arm's distance away from a bookcase, or any other flat stable object of at least shoulder height. Let arms hang loosely at the sides (Figure 12-3a).

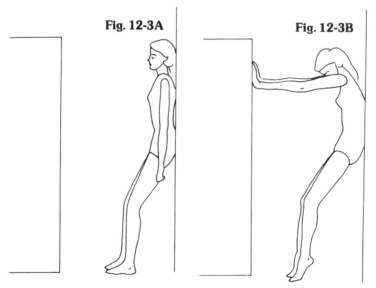

Fig. 12-3A   Fig. 12-3B

Movements:

1. On an inhale push palms of hands into bookcase opposite you; rise up on your toes and press small of back firmly into the wall, dropping head forward and rounding shoulders and upper back (Figure 12-3b).
2. Exhale; relax arms and body without letting go of the wall, and lower heels back to floor, bending knees. Return hands and upper back to starting position.

The sitting self-massage

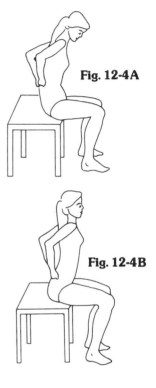

Fig. 12-4A

Starting position:
Sit on a chair with legs comfortably apart.

Note: *Never massage directly on the vertebrae of the spine.*

Movements:

1. Clench hands into fists and place them behind you as high as you can reach on either side of your spine (Figure 12-4a).
2. On an inhale (or as the contraction begins) arch your back (tilting pelvis down) and slowly but forcefully move fists down to the base of your spine (Figure 12-4b).

Fig. 12-4B

3. Exhale and move fists back up to starting position while tilting pelvis back up.
4. Repeat for as long as you like, in a slow, smooth flowing motion.

Tip: *A few drops of Olbas oil rubbed into the lower back, especially at the sacrum, has a soothing, warming effect which can be very relieving for back labor; this promotes warmth, which in turn loosens up muscles and ligaments.*

CLEARING THE NASAL AIR PASSAGES

To offset the "stuffed nose" typical of advanced pregnancy (because of the natural swelling of mucus membranes), and make breathing easier, dab a few drops of Olbas oil or Vicks VapoRub on your nostrils from time to time. Don't use nose drops; they could possibly have a slowing-down effect on your contractions.

THE SITTING-BIRTH DANCE

In between contractions you might try helping nature along by doing the sitting-birth dance. This relaxed side-to-side swaying of the hips has a limbering-up effect on the pelvic ligaments (which need to give considerably during labor) and helps shuffle the baby farther down into the pelvis, where it can aid in the dilation of the cervix by pressing against it from the inside.

To start, sit squarely on your seat bones near the edge of a firm chair, with legs comfortably apart, feet flat on the floor, and hands resting limply on the chair or falling freely at the sides. Then relax, letting your spine hollow naturally at the waist and gently shift your weight and pelvis from side to side, in a smooth almost effortless motion, bringing your head to move freely with each twist of the spine (Figure 12-5).

If your contractions seem to be letting up instead of growing stronger or if labor progresses very slowly (either at home or at the hospital), try to intensify your contractions by putting some swerve into your "dance": Tilt your pelvis down and swing it around in a circular movement as if you were doing a slow motion belly dance. Continue to dance on and off between contractions for several minutes or until you have achieved the desired effect, always stopping to lean forward and breathe calmly over each oncoming contraction.

As weird as this sitting belly dance may seem to the Western mind, it's certainly simpler, and safer, than speeding up labor with drugs!

Note: *Never do the more lively version of the sitting-birth dance continuously before your due date.*

Fig. 12-5

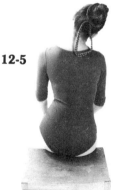

THE RELAXING BATH

One natural way of taking the edge off labor pains, and stimulating your circulation (which means getting a good flow of blood to the uterus), is to wallow leisurely in a hot bath before leaving for the hospital. As shocking as this may seem to some, there are doctors and midwives all over Europe who believe bathing during first-stage labor can be beneficial, as long as the membranes remain intact. Opinions vary, so *check with your doctor.* If you should decide on the bath, be sure to take it only in your own sparkling clean tub when someone else is at home. Also, don't lock the bathroom door, don't let the water run cold, and don't stay in longer than 20 minutes, as contractions seem to melt away in the warmth of the water (despite their mounting intensity) and you want to keep an eye on their progress. Occasionally it takes a while for contractions to set in again after the bath. Don't worry. If they're true labor contractions they will soon return.

TIME TO LEAVE

It's often hard to know just when it's time to leave for the hospital. Most doctors and hospitals have their own set of rules to guide you, but babies are notorious for breaking rules. So use some common sense. Trust your intuition. And consider the following: the length of time between contractions; the duration of the contractions themselves; whether or not the membranes have ruptured or leaked; whether there was a "show" of blood-stained mucus; and, of course, how far you are from the hospital.

Stay calm and don't be overly concerned about getting there too late or too soon. More often than not the mother is the first one to know when it's time to go.

COPING AT THE HOSPITAL

THE ENEMA

Usually an enema is given upon admission to the hospital. While the enema is taking effect, you'll have the discomfort of stomach cramps in addition to your contractions.

To help you cope with both, ask the nurse for a chair, place it backwards in front of you, and lean forward to rest your folded arms and head on the chair back (see Figure 12-6). In

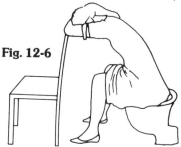

Fig. 12-6

this more comfortable position breathe over your contractions, using either deep, full breathing or one of the first two forms of graduated breathing. In between contractions you might try doing the birth dance, especially if you've been told your contractions are weak and ineffectual.

GETTING ON WITH LABOR

Once you've settled down comfortably to relax and breathe over your contractions don't let anything or anyone distract you. Most of all, *don't let anything upset you.* Don't fret over minor details or the seemingly unfriendly attitude of some nurse. Take it in your stride. Accept the situation. Adapt to your circumstances.

Keep your priorities clearly in view: your first job is to relax, and that comes from within, not from without. Remember, the ability to relax emotionally and physically during labor, regardless of all prevailing conditions, improves *your* chances for an easier, calmer, more bearable childbirth.

So just concentrate on letting go-o- and breathing over your contractions, and leave all the little aggravations that almost always arise to your husband.* Let him fend for you. He's your best public relations man. With a firm but charming smile he can usually cope with any resistance on the part of

---

*Today, finding a hospital that allows fathers to participate during labor and delivery has become easier, although it may mean traveling somewhat farther from home. Nevertheless, it pays. Just having someone you love near you during childbirth is psychologically very beneficial. So plan ahead. Shop around carefully before choosing a hospital.

the nursing staff. (Fortunately, the peacefulness manifested by the deep, trancelike relaxation eventually wins the admiration and cooperation of the attending medical personnel.)

If you do allow yourself to become frustrated and angry, you will be hurting only yourself and your baby. No matter how justified you may be, blaming the hospital or the doctor (of your choice!) will not compensate for the unnecessary pain you'll be causing yourself by your own mental tension.

THOSE LAST FEW CONTRACTIONS

At some point near the end of the first stage (*especially if labor is being speeded up with drugs*), a woman who has been managing beautifully all along may experience an unexpected moment of crisis when the sudden stepped-up intensity of her contractions seems to threaten her equanimity; relaxation hangs in the balance, and there's a feeling of restlessness, even an urge to get up and do something.

If this should happen to you, take it as a sign that you've almost reached your goal—your baby is about to arrive—and make an all-out last effort to relax. Concentrate more intensely on letting go, feeling heavy, and sinking down deeper and deeper into your bed. The crisis will soon pass.

Remember, except for possibly changing to an all-fours position, to be physically active at this late stage could cause you much unnecessary pain. You simply can't be fully relaxed if you're fidgeting, talking, or grasping the guards of a hospital bed. Tension has a way of spreading, especially under stress. So instead of gritting your teeth and squeezing your husband's hand, let your mouth and body go limp and heavy. *Think* of your baby making its way farther down through your body, and concentrate on your breathing. You'll soon find yourself back in control.

Chapter Thirteen

POINTERS FOR FATHERS

Aside from the definite psychological lift your presence affords the mother during labor and delivery there are a number of ways in which you can help.

IN THE LABOR ROOM

Right from the start you can make relaxation just so much easier for the laboring mother by turning off any glaring, warm, overhead lights and leaving only one small light burning. If there is a window in the room, open it to let in some fresh (oxygen rich) air and draw the shades during the daytime. It also helps to close the door, when possible, or else leave it only slightly ajar. If the labor "room" constitutes only a small cubicle set apart by drapes, draw them closed to shut out any disturbing noises and light as much as possible.

In short, do everything you can to ensure that the labor room is dim, peaceful, and airy. Fortunately you are not likely to run into any opposition by all this. After all, who could reasonably object to a mother's turning down the lights and going to "sleep" during labor? Nevertheless, hospitals are unpredictable, so discuss your plans with your doctor well in advance. It's always best to have "doctor's approval" to fall back on, just in case.

EASING BACK-LABOR

For most women, contractions felt in the lower back are the most trying. To help ease back-labor many Swiss midwives and doctors give the laboring mother a counterpressure back massage. In the absence of such professional assistance, the father or any other "helper" present should do the following:

Keeping fingers side by side and straight with thumbs crossed (Figure 13-1), mold your hands to the mother's back, just there where it hurts. She can show you where by pointing with her hand (the one resting behind her).

During the contraction, lean forward, bending elbows out at the sides, and use the force of your weight to apply a firm, *even* pressure with your flat hands as the mother breathes over her contraction, using graduated breathing and gently presses her back into your hands. Don't shove or dig your fingers into her skin. A firm, steady, counterpressure is all that is needed—not a full-fledged massage!

Note: *Done on a bare back, it helps to pour some Olbas oil into the palms of your hands before you start.*

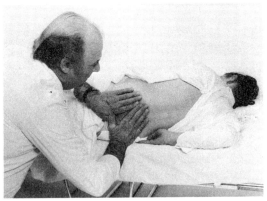

Fig. 13-1

AVOIDING A WELL-INTENDED ERROR

Unless your wife has developed the neuromuscular control of a yogi, she will not be able to tense her hand in order to grasp yours, without tensing up in other areas as well. The human body is simply too well interconnected for that.

In the light of this fact many Swiss midwives are trained to respond to a woman's reaching out for a hand to hold during labor or clenching her hands into fists by gently but firmly opening the mother's closed hand and stroking palm and fingers in a light upward motion. This soothing, stroking of the hand is very calming and conveys the message that someone is there who cares, without interfering with conscious relaxation. To learn how it's done study Figures 13-2a, 13-2b, and 13-2c.

Note: *Once you notice the mother regaining her calm, lower her hand gently to the bed. Holding it longer might disturb her deep conscious relaxation.*

Fig. 13-2A   **Fig. 13-2B**

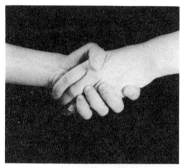 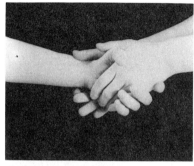

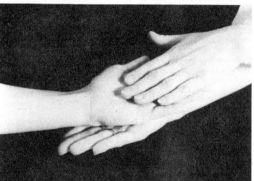

Fig. 13-2C

ACTING AS BREATHING COACH

Besides acquainting yourself with deep-conscious relaxation and the pushing technique, it pays to learn how to low-pant.

Although your wife may never need to low-pant during first-stage labor, she may very well need it at the start of the second stage to fight her urge to push. In which case you could be of invaluable assistance if you are able to help her keep up her rhythm by clapping your hands in time to the usual low-panting beat: 1-2-3-4-5-6 and then giving a clearly audible, "Shhh-huuh," to accentuate the quick "exchange of air."

HELPING DURING "TRANSITION"

If you notice the mother suddenly becoming restless, fidgeting with her hands or feet, grasping the guards of the bed, or showing any other signs of tension, try to help her regain her calm and control by reminding her in a soft, soothing voice to let go and sink down deeper into her bed. You will not have time to go through the whole deep-conscious relaxation text, so concentrate on the main points: Tell her to relax her mouth and to *feel* how vast and hollow it is and how heavy her tongue grows. From there, go on to the upper shoulder and the upper thigh, telling her to let them go-o-, allowing the entire contents of her breastcage and pelvis to spill out, down into the bed. If she has practiced often before, this should be enough to bring her back into a state of deep, conscious relaxation. But, of course, a word of encouragement is also helpful. Let her know that the extra pressure she feels is probably the baby moving farther down in her pelvis and that she must be near the end of dilation. She probably is. So don't wait too long to notify the nurse or whoever is in charge of the change in her contractions.

HELPING IN THE DELIVERY ROOM

There is more to being a Father-in-the-Delivery-Room than donning a white cap and gown and coaching your wife to push hard—provided you've come prepared. Right from the start you may be needed to help her low-pant through those first few pushing contractions, when she must keep herself back from pushing too soon. When she's given the green light to bear down you can act as her coach, calling out the movements in turn: deep sign, head back, gulp, etc.; cheering her on to push in the direction of the birth canal; and if you like, pushing right along with her. Just don't get carried away. Your pushes won't help as much as your ability to spot any faults in hers. So keep your eyes open. If she's pushing full force yet seems distraught, looks exasperated, and wears a pained, frenzied expression (complete with knotted brow, deep frown, and popped veins), then she's pushing all wrong and needs help—quickly! Not because she's in pain. Poor, ineffectual pushing is not painful (although it may seem that way to the untrained eye), but it is distressing. And the frustration of working so hard without getting anywhere can be agonizing. Here's where you can help. Not with cheers of, "Keep it up. You're doing great!" but by keeping calm and pinpointing what's causing all the trouble. Check if she:

> Forgets to take a deep sigh at the start of her contraction.
> Fails to make a faint gasping sound as she "catches" a mouthful of air. If she doesn't then she is not inhaling enough.
> Pushes with an open mouth.
> Keeps her lips closed, makes low grunting throaty sounds, puffs out her cheeks and grows red in the face. All of which indicate that she hasn't fully closed the "trap" in her throat and is pushing up into her head instead of downward and forward in the direction of the birth passage.
> Fails to curl head and shoulders forward.
> Draws her elbows (and possibly even her knees) together, or keeps her elbows down on the table instead of lifting them up and out at the sides.

If she's doing any or all of the above, don't despair. It's not too late to step in and re-educate her, right then and there on the delivery table. Women in advanced labor have an uncanny knack for learning how to push—but getting through to them can be difficult. Remember your wife is likely to be too engrossed in her own frantic struggle to push to pay any attention to you or your advice—at first. It may take some doing to get your message across, but it can be done! Start by telling her exactly what's wrong. If, for instance, she's pushing with an open mouth she is probably unaware of it. She *thinks* her mouth is closed. So tell her, gently but firmly, "Your mouth is open. Purse your lips." If that doesn't work, take a quick "gulp" yourself and purse your lips. Exaggerate! Make sure that she sees. Don't get discouraged if she doesn't seem to comprehend at first. Keep on trying and she'll catch on. When she does, go on to correct the next error (if any), and then the next, until she's pushing just right. When she is, you'll both notice the difference (and possibly even the results). After that, it shouldn't take more than a few good satisfying pushes for your baby to be born.

Chapter Fourteen

FINISHING TOUCHES

THE THIRD STAGE

As soon as the baby is born, the third stage of labor sets in and placenta and membranes have to be expelled. This usually occurs within minutes (especially if you receive an injection of oxytocin), but it can take considerably longer. In any case, it does not hurt but comes slithering out (noisily) with little more than one half-strength push. Now your work is done, but not your doctor's. He still has to examine the placenta and membranes, and if an episiotomy was performed or a laceration occurred, he has some sewing to do before he can leave.

While procedures do vary from country to country and even from one hospital to the next in the same city, in most Swiss hospitals today the mother is free (and often encouraged) to touch, hold, and stroke her newborn baby even before it receives its first soothing, warm bath. Once it is washed and dressed, she may very well nurse it right there on the delivery table—a procedure which helps stimulate the expulsion of the placenta.

Before the midwife (whose sphere of work in Switzerland is usually curtailed to assisting the doctor in charge) hurries off to leave the new "family" to themselves, she usually helps the mother freshen up by giving her a sponge bath, helping her into her own nightgown, bringing her make-up case, toothbrush, and toothpaste, complete with a cup of water and a basin. Then comes the coffee, cocoa, or tea that adds that perfect last touch to an already blissful moment and makes her feel like a queen—or so it always seemed to me.

SUMMING UP NATURAL CHILDBIRTH PREPARATION: WAS IT WORTH IT?

Preparing for a truly natural birth takes time, effort and a certain amount of stamina, all qualities which make for good parenting as well. But, when you experience the special thrill and challenge of a natural childbirth, you'll know, beyond a doubt, that it was worth it all. In years to come, the knowledge that you were able to cope and bring the months of your pregnancy to a safe and gratifying conclusion for both you and your baby will give you untold satisfaction. Granted, you may never be able to pinpoint the advantages and say for certain, "Because of my efforts he (or she) is just so much better developed, or just so much calmer." But neither will you ever have cause to wonder, should anything go amiss, if some childbirth drug or instrument was to blame.

Surely the many disquieting reports of recent studies being made on the effects of childbirth drugs on the newborn, plus the increased likelihood of forceps delivery whenever any of the popular regional anesthetics (conduction blocks) are used, should be cause enough to work toward a natural childbirth. Even in the absence of tangible proof, it stands to reason that if the trauma of birth is that all-important first step in life, then surely a natural, *calm* childbirth is a first step taken in the right direction.

IV

RECOVERY

Chapter Fifteen

RECOVERY ROOM EXERCISES

You're no longer pregnant and you're not sick, but you're not quite your old self either. How could you be? For months your body has been building up to the climactic event of birth. Now it needs time to readjust and return to its pre-pregnant state. And you need time to recuperate from the emotional and physical stress of birth. After all, you've just started on the road to recovery and there's still a long way to go before you arrive. For that reason, you should start your postpartum program as soon as you can.

As soon as possible after birth start with the following simple exercises to stir up your slowed-down circulation and guard against possible circulatory complications. Do them once or even twice before finally settling down for that first deep, well-deserved sleep.

Chest breathing exercise

Movements:
1. Place one hand lightly on your chest and inhale slowly, breathing in towards your hand. Feel your chest expand as your hand rises.
2. Then exhale very slowly and very thoroughly, causing hand to sink back down as chest deflates.
3. Repeat once. Then pause to rest, breathing naturally.

The abdominal up-sweep

Movements:
1. Slowly draw a full-deep breath in, inflating belly, midriff, and chest.

2. Exhale very thoroughly, expelling every trace of air from your lungs as you pull tummy tightly in (drawing navel to spine) and tighten the beltlike muscles of your waist (which cross over the abdomen from side to side).

3. Then, when your lungs are empty, lift and suck in your abdomen so that your midriff appears hollow directly under your ribs (Figure 15-1).

4. Hold. Await the need to inhale before inhaling slowly and deeply, filling your lungs zestfully.

5. Repeat once. Then pause and relax.

Tip: *The "sucking in" action is done by going through the motions of inhaling without actually breathing in any air.*

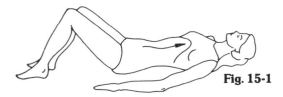

Fig. 15-1

The leg-press

Movements:

1. Keeping legs straight and pressed together, with ankles bent back sharply, tense buttocks, pelvic floor and legs, bringing heels to rise slightly off the bed (Figure 15-2).

2. Hold the tension for a count of ten. Then relax and breathe deeply. Repeat once.

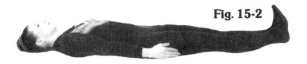

Fig. 15-2

The lying-down run

Note: *Gradually accelerate all of the following movements and then slow them down again before stopping.*

Starting position:
Keeping arms close at the sides, bend them at the elbows, lifting hands off the bed, and press elbows down into your bed.

Movements:
1. Keeping elbows pressed down and close to chest, alternately clench hands into fists and open them wide, spreading fingers out with such intensity that palms and fingers turn white (Figure 15-3a). Repeat about 8 times, always quickening and then slowing down your tempo.
2. Shake hands up and down (Figures 15-3b and 15-3c), in and out, and around in circles, clockwise and counterclockwise. Do this several times, making sure to keep elbows pressed down at the sides until you are finished exercising your hands.

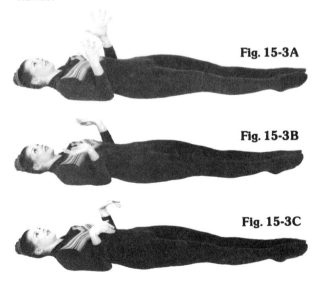

Fig. 15-3A

Fig. 15-3B

Fig. 15-3C

3. Then bend and stretch toes several times and, keeping heels on bed, move feet up and down, in and out, and around in circles, in both directions.
4. Now, keeping both elbows and heels on the bed, work both hands and feet simultaneously: first bend and stretch fingers and toes and then move hands and feet briskly up and down, in and out, and around in circles, clockwise and counterclockwise, for approximately 30 seconds.
5. Then shake hands and feet vigorously to de-tense.
6. Rest and breathe deeply, according to your own natural breathing rhythm. If you place a hand on your heart you should feel it beating wildly as if after a good invigorating run.

Chapter Sixteen
THE WAY BACK

Don't be lulled into a false sense of complacency if you find you're in better shape than the woman lying in the next bed. Your work is still not quite done, although you are closer to your goal than most postpartum mothers. Despite prenatal care and exercise, your muscles and even your skin have been stretched for months, and they need a chance to recuperate. During the next few weeks you will notice a marked improvement in your figure, especially if you nudge nature along by exercising.

Be careful though. Avoid putting too much strain on your weakened muscles too soon. Even if you feel up to it, don't do any strenuous exercise during the first postpartum days. Muscles are living elastic; if you stretch them too thin, they may lose their ability to recoil all the way.

In Switzerland, hospitals generally provide their postpartum patients with the services of a qualified physical therapist. Following are some typical exercises in this step-by-step program. Besides aiding in the natural process of rehabilitation, they also improve circulation and help to avoid the circulatory complications which can surface during those first few postpartum days.

POSTPARTUM GUIDELINES

Like pregnancy, the postpartum period has its guidelines. Stick to them rigidly, in order to cut down on fatigue and protect your strained muscles from further harm, especially the rectus muscles running up and down your abdomen. During pregnancy these normally taut, straight muscles were forced apart, and it will take some time for them to return to their usual side-by-side position. Until that happens, use them sparingly.

1. When exercising, always open a window; remove pillows and covers if you are lying in bed.
2. When sitting up or getting out of bed, always bend your knees and roll to one side, just as you did during pregnancy.
3. When lying in a supine position, never lift or lower both your outstretched legs simultaneously.
4. To draw knees up at a 45-degree angle, bend first one and then the other—never both at once.
5. Never curl your head and torso forward all the way. Pulling yourself up too far could cause the stretched rectus muscles to bend, thereby widening the gap between them.
6. Don't do any squatting exercises until after your final postpartum examination.
7. In addition to doing the early postpartum exercises, make it a habit always to stop the flow in midstream two or three times whenever you urinate—even if it hurts. This helps stimulate circulation in the area, and it may even aid the healing process.

EARLY POSTPARTUM EXERCISES

Basic starting positions:

Position A: Lie flat on your back with legs stretched out straight on the bed and arms either extended sideways or down at the sides.

Position B: Lie on back with knees together, bent at a 45-degree angle, and feet flat on the bed. Arms are naturally at the sides or extended sideways at shoulder level.

THE FIRST POSTPARTUM DAY

In addition to doing the recovery room exercises several times during the day, do the following exercises at least once.

The chest-expander

Starting position:
Position A with arms down at the sides.

Movements:
1. Inhale slowly and deeply as you slide arms sideways and up as far as you can reach, inscribing a wide half-circle with each arm.
2. Then exhale (on *sssss*) and smoothly slide arms back down to starting position.
3. Repeat three times.

The head curl

Starting position:
Position A with arms along sides.

Movements:
1. Exhale and raise head to touch chin to chest. Hold a moment.
2. Then return head to starting position and inhale deeply.
3. Repeat 5 times.

The lazy pelvic tilt

Starting position:
Position B with arms at the sides.

Movements:
1. Inhale and tilt pelvis down, arching small of back and relaxing abdominal and pelvic floor muscles.
2. Exhale and tilt pelvis up, pulling tummy firmly in toward spine, pressing small of back to floor and tucking seat under.
3. Repeat 6-8 times.
4. Relax and limber up by swinging spine gently back and forth. (See page 38).

The knee press

Starting position:
Position B with arms at the sides.

Movements:
1. On an exhale pull tummy firmly in, press small of back into bed and squeeze knees together, tensing seat and pelvic floor muscles at the same time. Hold for a count of 6.
2. Then inhale and relax slowly.
3. Repeat twice.

Elevated foot work

Starting position:
Position B with arms naturally along sides.

Movements:
1. Exhale and draw tummy firmly in, pressing small of back farther into bed and pressing knees slightly together.
2. Keeping knees pressed together, inhale, kick calf of one leg up straight, with toes pointed and tense raised leg from top to bottom (Figure 16-1).
3. Breathing naturally, bend and stretch toes of raised leg several times. Then move the foot up and down; in and out; and around in circles in both directions.
4. Drop calf of raised leg, letting it fall back down into starting position.
5. Relax and breathe naturally.
6. Repeat once with your other leg.

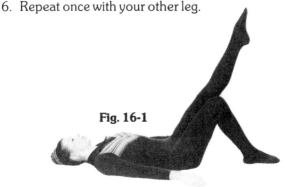

Fig. 16-1

To help your uterus return to a good position as quickly as possible, always end your postpartum exercise routine for the day by turning over and resting with one or two pillows under your belly (Figure 16-2). Use this pillow-under-belly position often during the next few weeks, even while sleeping.

Fig. 16-2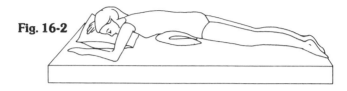

THE SECOND POSTPARTUM DAY
In addition to those exercises practiced on the first postpartum day, do the following:

The body bounce
Starting position:
Position A with legs crossed at ankles and arms along sides with palms of hands flat on the bed for better balance.

Movements:
1. On an exhale tense legs and pelvis very hard and slowly bounce your bottom and most of your upper body off the bed, resting your weight entirely on shoulders and lower heels. Use hands only for balance. See Figure 16-3.
2. Bounce slightly up and down 3-4 times without touching bottom.
3. Then slowly lower yourself back down to starting position.
4. Repeat 2-3 times.

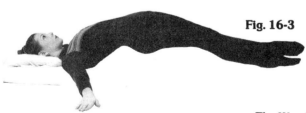

Fig. 16-3

The double knee roll

Starting position:
Position B with arms straight out at the sides at shoulder level, holding on to the sides of your bed.

Movements:
1. Keeping shoulders and arms down on the bed, gently drop both knees to the right as you inhale, touching right knee to bed and turning your head to the left (Figure 16-4).
2. With your next breath out press small of back to floor, pulling tummy in, and swing bent knees up to starting position.
3. Relax small of back and repeat exercise to the left as you inhale.
4. Swing legs smoothly from side to side 4 more times, always taking care to press small of back to bed as you swing knees up.

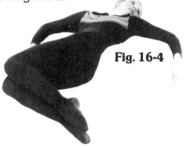

Fig. 16-4

The bent-leg lift

Starting position:
Position A with arms naturally along sides.

Movements:
1. Pull tummy firmly in, press small of back to bed, and slowly draw right knee up to chest.
2. Flex ankle (Figure 16-5a).

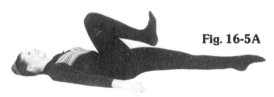

Fig. 16-5A

3. With heel leading, stretch raised leg out, diagonally (Figure 16-5b).

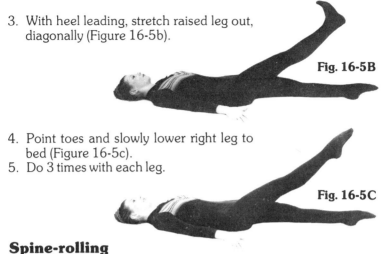

Fig. 16-5B

4. Point toes and slowly lower right leg to bed (Figure 16-5c).
5. Do 3 times with each leg.

Fig. 16-5C

Spine-rolling

See page 92 for instructions.

Finish off by turning around and resting quietly with a pillow under your stomach.

THE THIRD POSTPARTUM DAY

Add the following to yesterday's exercise routine (including the recovery room exercises).

The sliding-arm head curl

Substitute for the head curl

Starting position:
Position A with arms at sides and with ankles and wrists flexed so that toes and fingers point up to ceiling.
Movements:
1. On an exhale, pull tummy sharply in toward spine and curl head and shoulders slightly forward off the bed, touching chin to chest and sliding outstretched arms forward along your bed (Figure 16-6).

Fig. 16-6

2. Hold a moment.
3. Inhale and slowly uncurl, drawing head, shoulders, and arms back to starting position.
4. Repeat twice for today, gradually working up to 6 times as the days go by and your strength increases.

The side-twisting body curl

Starting position:
Position B with left arm crossed over to the right and hand resting, palm down, on the outside of your right hip.

Movements:
1. Exhale slowly (sssss), drawing tummy in and pressing small of back into bed, and reach left hand forward and downward to touch the bed; curling head and left shoulder up off the bed as you twist to the right (Figure 16-7).

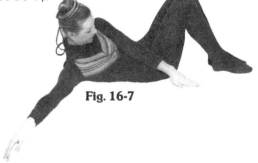

Fig. 16-7

2. Then hold and inhale.
3. Exhale and slowly return to starting position. Relax and breathe naturally.
4. Alternating arms, repeat twice on each side.

Waistline tucks

See page 75 for instructions.

End by resting in the usual pillow-under-tummy position.

THE FOURTH POSTPARTDUM DAY
Add the following to yesterday's exercise routine:

The one-legged twist
See page 73 for instructions. Do steps 1 through 3.

Now roll over on your stomach and rest with a pillow under your tummy.

THE FIFTH POSTPARTUM DAY
Add the following to yesterday's routine.

The arm-leg swing
Starting position:
Lie on your back with legs comfortably apart and arms stretched out at the sides at shoulder level.

Movements:
1. Simultaneously swing right leg up high and swing left arm up and across to the right, raising head and left shoulder off the bed and twisting torso to the right as you cross swinging arm with swinging leg at hip level (Figure 16-8).

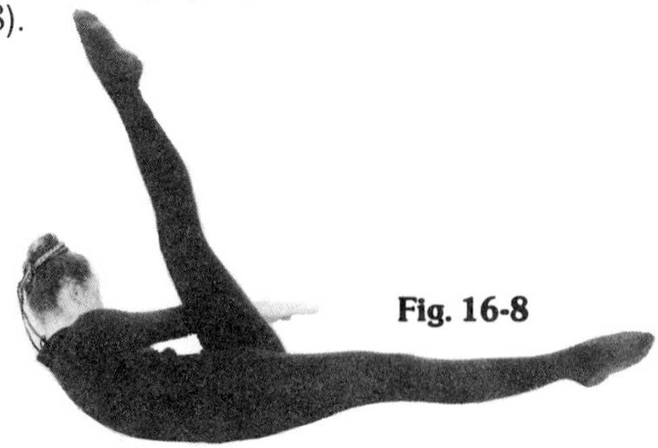

Fig. 16-8

2. Then without stopping, swing leg and arm back down to starting position, lowering head and left shoulder back to bed.
3. Repeat with right arm and left leg. Then do it 4 more times nonstop, alternately crossing arms and legs quickly to give you more momentum.

Air lifts

Starting position:
Lie on your stomach, your head cradled in your arms and your legs side by side. Place a pillow under your midriff to relieve pressure on your breasts, and anchor your feet to the bed by placing your toes between the mattress and the bed post. Better still, have someone hold them down, if possible.

Movements:
1. Tense body from head to toe and slowly lift arms, head, and torso off the bed, stretching arms out and up in front (Figure 16-9).
2. Hold for a moment. Then lower slowly.
3. Repeat twice.

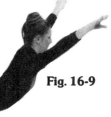

Fig. 16-9

Finish off by resting in the usual pillow-under-tummy position.

THE SIXTH POSTPARTUM DAY
Add to yesterday's routine:

The thigh-bump

Starting position:
Lie on your stomach with one leg stretched out on the bed and one bent behind you with calf raised and toes pointing to ceiling. For comfort, place a pillow under your midriff and cradle your head in your arms.

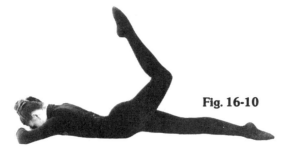

Fig. 16-10

Movements:
1. Keeping hip bones pressed to bed, raise your bent leg up and down several times (Figure 16-10).
2. Repeat with your other leg.

Finish off by resting in the usual position.

ADVANCED POSTPARTUM EXERCISES

From here on you can continue doing the sixth postpartum day exercise routine until all vaginal bleeding has stopped and you've been given your doctor's okay to start a more vigorous program.

Once you are up and about, you can leave recovery room exercises out of your daily routine, except for the up-sweep (p. 187) which should be done every day, preferably in the morning when you wake up and again at night before falling asleep.

THE POSTPARTUM FOLLOW-UP

If after your postpartum visit you're not quite satisfied with the shape you're in—or even if you are—don't stop now!

Clinically speaking, the postpartum period lasts six to eight weeks, but complete rehabilitation of lax pelvic joints and abdominal muscles can take from three to twelve months. With concentrated, vigorous exercises, you can do much to help the forces of nature with your own energetic attack on stomach, thighs, and "undercarriage."

In Switzerland most women attend special postnatal exercise classes for several months after their postpartum examination. It will be worth your while to find a good, vigorous exercise class of your own.

If you are nursing, don't expect to see the true results of your pre- and postnatal efforts until after you've stopped breastfeeding. During lactation your body naturally retains more fluid and fat, although it is actually burning up more calories.

EPILOGUE:
LOOKING AHEAD

The rewards of your prenatal and postnatal training should be felt long after your baby is born. You may notice it in the lightness of your walk, the ease of your movements, and the self-confidence and vitality that come from being in tune with your body. In fact, by the end of your childbearing cycle (pregnancy—birth—lactation), much of what you have learned about relaxation, breathing, and physical fitness may have become an integral part of your way of life.

Having attained a certain level of physical awareness, you may find that you can't turn all the way back to your pre-pregnancy ways. Taking care of yourself is habit-forming. It takes a certain effort—like brushing your teeth after every meal—but once you're used to it you don't feel quite right without it.

Which is all to the best—now that you've joined the ranks of motherhood. Within the next few weeks you're bound to discover that full-deep breathing and relaxation are lifesaving techniques, and that some form of regular exercise— whether it be swimming, jogging, or gymnastics—is indispensable when it comes to coping with the everyday stress and exhaustion of being mother, wife, and woman.

In short, pregnant or not, a relaxed, vital body is sunshine for your soul: it radiates warmth and energy and makes everything brighter.

INDEX